Dental Management

of

Ap

Au

Dental Management of the Handicapped: *Approaches for Dental Auxiliaries*

BRIAN MARK LANGE, Ph.D.

Assistant Professor
University of Nebraska Medical Center
College of Dentistry
Lincoln, Nebraska

BEVERLY MORSE ENTWISTLE, R.D.H., M.P.H.

Assistant Professor
University of Colorado: School of Dentistry
and the J.F.K. Child Development Center
Denver, Colorado

LAURETTE F. LIPSON, M.N.Ed.

Professor and Chairman
Department of Educational Services
Baylor College of Dentistry
Dallas, Texas

Lea & Febiger • 1983 • Philadelphia

Lea & Febiger
600 S. Washington Square
Philadelphia, PA 19106
U.S.A.

Library of Congress Cataloging in Publication Data

Lange, Brian Mark.
Dental management of the handicapped.

Includes index.
1. Handicapped—Dental care. 2. Dental auxiliary personnel. I. Entwistle, Beverly Morse. II. Lipson, Laurette F. III. Title. [DNLM: 1. Dental care for handicapped. 2. Dental auxiliaries. WU 29 L269d] RK55.H28L36 1983 617.6'00880816 82-23939 ISBN 0-8121-0884-1

PRINTED IN THE UNITED STATES OF AMERICA

Print Number: 3 2 1

PREFACE

Recommendations for curriculum guidelines for Dentistry for the Handicapped, developed in 1980 by a joint committee of the American Association of Dental Schools and the National Foundation of Dentistry for the Handicapped, signaled the beginning of a new era in dental education. The curriculum guidelines are the culmination of several years of effort by professionals representing several dental schools and organizations interested in educating dental students in special patient care. At present, several dental schools and hospital programs offer a variety of didactic and clinical experiences in the management of handicapped persons.

As interest in the care and treatment of the handicapped has grown, the dental profession has responded by developing texts to assist in this educational endeavor. The texts, as well as other dental literature, recommend a team approach to the dental treatment of handicapped persons. The team is generally described as consisting of the dentist, dental hygienist, dental assistant, receptionist, and/or office manager. Roles of the various team members, however, are not further delineated.

Recently, the Dental Hygiene Section of the American Association of Dental Schools recognized the need for a formalized educational approach to treating special patients. Workshops were given for dental hygiene educators in 1981 and 1982. In addition, a committee was established to develop curricular guidelines specifically pertaining to the dental hygienist's role with handicapped persons.

The intent of this book is to help fill a void in dental auxiliary education in the area of special patient care. The text is designed as an instructional manual for the student and as a reference manual for the practicing dental auxiliary. Several commonly occurring handicapping conditions are defined and described in terms of incidence, physical manifestations, and etiology. General medical and educational approaches are described, as well as psychosocial implications of the handicapping conditions. Special attention is devoted to implications for dental management, such as identifying and eliminating potential barriers to care and approaches to gathering and utilizing patient data for planning and counseling. Additionally, techniques for providing care, including problems that one should anticipate or prevent, treatment adaptations, and expected oral manifestations are explored. The development of realistic preventive programs is a major focus. Problem-solving situations in various formats are included at the conclusion of each chapter to challenge the reader to integrate and apply the information.

Three recurring themes are woven through each chapter: the concept of normalization, behavior management, and the team approach to dental treatment of handicapped patients.

The concept of "normalization," as used in the text, refers to the interaction strategies used to communicate with and treat handicapped patients. Specifically, normalization of dental treatment requires that handicapped individuals be managed along with all other patients, making allowances only for the limitations that the handicapping condition places upon the individual.

Behavioral management strategies are presented within the context of the simulated patient settings and scenarios. The behavioral strategies take the form of suggested tasks for members of the dental team and recommendations for how to encourage patients and significant others to develop and improve oral hygiene skills.

The team approach is emphasized to allow full development of the role of each person involved in providing oral health care and to maximize the normalization concept for the handicapped individual.

Whereas other texts primarily focus on the child patient, this text will consider the entire age spectrum. Dental hygienists and dental assistants are encouraged to use their skills in these vital areas to ensure that handicapped persons receive comprehensive dental care in the most optimal, dignified setting.

Lincoln, NE — B.M. Lange
Denver, CO — B.M. Entwistle
Dallas, TX — L.F. Lipson

ACKNOWLEDGEMENTS

The authors wish to express gratitude to those who contributed information to this book: Marilyn Greb, R.P.T., Craig Hospital, Englewood, Colorado, for her input on spinal injuries; John Coke, D.D.S., University of Colorado School of Dentistry, for his input on arthritis; Jody Neal Rees, R.D.H., R.D., M.S., Denver, Colorado for input on dietary and preventive considerations and her personal support.

We would also like to acknowledge: Kim Theesen for his drawing of the illustrations; Larry Sheffield for his photographic work; and Joan Hamilton for her usual outstanding job of typing.

Two individuals played a bigger role in the development of this book than they realize. John F. Simon, Jr., D.D.S., M.S.D., University of Nebraska Medical Center, and Paul Casamassimo, D.D.S., M.S., University of Colorado School of Dentistry, have not only provided professional and personal support, they have also provided unique contributions to the development and application of theories behind individualized care and preventive programs for handicapped persons.

B.M.L.
B.M.E.
L.F.L.

CONTENTS

Chapter 1
INTRODUCTION

DEFINITION OF HANDICAPPED

The term "handicapped" is used as an all-encompassing word to describe a group of individuals who exhibit a variety of debilitating conditions. A multitude of legal, educational, and medical definitions have been used to describe the term and its various subcategories. Sections 503 and 504 of the Rehabilitation Act of 1973 defines as handicapped any person who:

1) has a physical or mental impairment which substantially limits one or more major life activities such as caring for one's self, performing manual tasks, walking, seeing, hearing, speaking, breathing, learning and working.
2) has a record of such an impairment (has a history of or has been misclassified as having a condition that limits major life activities).
3) is regarded as having such an impairment.[1]

A person who is handicapped, therefore, may be labeled as such because of one condition or a variety of conditions involving medical, physical, mental, behavioral, sensory, or learning difficulties. The severity of these conditions varies from a minor abnormality that is not functionally significant to a severe impairment that creates total dependence. Individual responses and adaptations to these conditions also vary. Similarly, conditions are manifested differently throughout the various age spans.

Most of us have experienced temporary periods of being handicapped, either through illness or an accident. During these times we encounter the same problems as someone who has a record of impairment, but our overall outlook is probably less pessimistic or guarded because of the temporary nature of the disability.

EVOLUTION OF DENTAL CARE FOR THE HANDICAPPED

Dental literature pertaining to handicapped persons traditionally combined people with divergent disabilities into a homogeneous group, reportedly requiring significant changes in the provision of dental care. The evolution of dental care for these individuals can be described in four stages: (1) supervised neglect, (2) restraints and sedation, (3) specialized equipment, and (4) normalization. Each stage reflects the prevalent societal views of the time.

During the first stage many handicapped persons were denied their legal and civil rights, including the right to treatment. Dental treatment, if performed at all, was primarily reserved for emergency situations, particularly extreme pain and trauma. Tooth extractions dominated treatment planning. With the advent of more sophisticated restorative procedures and the development of dental clinics in institutionalized settings, the dental profession recognized its responsibility to provide more appropriate care. Most care during this period, although of higher quality, was delivered under abnormal conditions, with widespread use of general anesthesia, oral sedation, and physical restraints.

The early 1970s ushered in a national outcry against the general inhumane treatment of handicapped persons. Such practices as the indiscriminate use of physical restraints was declared a form of abuse. To facilitate the provision of dental treatment and maintenance of oral hygiene, numerous specialized techniques and equipment were designed for various types of handicapping conditions, including hydraulic wheelchair tilts, head stabilizers, and adapted toothbrushes. Dentistry for the handicapped became a dental subspecialty, characterized by a small group of dedicated professionals who possessed specialized skills and relied on specialized equipment and techniques.

During the 1970s the concepts of normalization and deinstitutionalization emerged as the themes of the time. Normalization, a process advanced by Nirje in Scandinavia and Wolfensberger in the United States, is defined as "making available to the mentally retarded, patterns and conditions of everyday life which are as close as possible to the norms and patterns of the mainstream of society."[2] The concept of normalization suggests that (1) services should be provided in a manner that makes individuals appear less different, (2) the similarity of individuals to other people, not their differences, should be emphasized, and (3) the values of society should be shaped to accept harmless differences in people.[3] The normalization process calls for introducing or reintegrating handicapped people into society, without sheltering them from the risks involved with daily experiences and decision making.

Implementation of Normalization. The broad concept of normalization was implemented through legislation, and programs for handicapped persons were developed to meet the goals of:

1. ensuring their legal and civil rights
2. receiving an appropriate education
3. increasing social skills and problem-solving abilities
4. increasing employment options and decreasing employer discrimination
5. ensuring a comprehensive network of community resources

An educational milestone occurred in 1975 when Congress passed the Education of All Handicapped Children Act (PL 94-142), which mandated local school districts to provide a free, appropriate education to all children, regardless of their disabilities. In addition, individual education plans for each child receiving special services were mandated to ensure teacher accountability and student progress.[4]

In 1977 the Secretary of Health, Education and Welfare (now Health and Human Services) approved regulations that led to the full implementation of Section 504 of the Rehabilitation Act of 1973. Discrimination against persons who have physical, mental or psychologic disabilities was thus deemed illegal.[5] The implementation of 504 called for the withholding of federal funds from any construction project that was not physically accessible to handicapped individuals.[6] People who were institutionalized or previously denied services were suddenly placed in a variety of living, learning, and working situations. A host of agencies and professionals emerged to meet the needs of these people (Table 1–1). Federal and private funding for such endeavors increased dramatically during this time.

Dental Curriculum Development Grants. Dental schools also benefited through curriculum development grants awarded to 11 schools in 1974 by the Robert Wood Johnson Foundation. The purpose of this funding effort was to educate future dentists in the care of handicapped patients with the anticipation that these dentists would integrate handicapped patients into their general dental practices.[7] Special teaching clinics were established at some of the schools, while others integrated handicapped patients into the regular clinics.[8] Students were taught to dispense with preconceived stereotypes and myths about handicapped people and to approach dental care from a more personalized perspective, emphasizing individualized treatment planning and providing treatment in the

TABLE 1–1. A Selection of Professional Resources for Handicapped Persons.

Services/Agencies	Professionals
Education	Physician
Advocacy	Psychologist
Health care	Special education teacher
Social services	Educational consultant
Mental health	Dental personnel
Residential	Physical therapist
Work training	Advocate
Employment	Social worker/Case worker
Legal support	Rehabilitation counselor
Habitation	Speech/Language therapist
Recreation	Dietician/Nutritionist
	Nurse
	Occupational therapist
	Recreation therapist

least restrictive setting for the patient. Normalization of dental care, then, has gradually emerged as a reality in the United States.

THE DENTAL TEAM CONCEPT

During the last decade significant changes have also occurred in the education and utilization of dental auxiliaries. With the emphasis in the 1970s on expanded duties, the team approach, and preventive dentistry, dental hygienists, dental assistants, and expanded function dental auxiliaries (EFDAs) have assumed increasing responsibilities for direct patient care, dental health education, and program planning.[9] The expanded responsibilities have also increased the variety of settings in which dental auxiliaries may engage in practice. These settings include, but are not limited to, hospitals, solo and group practices, public clinics, schools, universities, residential care facilities, and industry.

The role of auxiliaries will vary depending on the environment (i.e., hospital, school, solo practice), the goals of the team, and the management style of the team leader. Part of what unifies a team is working together to identify and adjust the individual roles each team member will fulfill. The dental hygienist and dental assistant often find themselves in a pivotal role when interacting with patients. In many instances, they set the tone for the dental experience and establish the first line of communication in the dental setting. This tone and line of communication take on a new meaning when the patient has a handicapping condition, and may make the difference between well-met dental needs for handicapped individuals or continued frustration for persons whose oral health needs often go unattended. It becomes critical for all members of the team to understand the causes of and problems related to handicapping conditions in order to plan and conduct a rewarding dental experience for the patient.

PATIENT MANAGEMENT STRATEGIES

Integrating the concept of normalization of handicapped patients into a regular dental practice requires that allowances be made only for the limitations that the handicapping condition places upon the individual. In preparing for and treating handicapped individuals, members of the dental health team must employ problem-solving/awareness strategies in relation to the patient and the handicapping condition if interaction and dental care are to be effective and satisfying for both the patient and the team members. These problem-solving/awareness strategies can be developed in four ways:

1. development of a patient condition profile
2. application of a problem-solving assessment technique
3. use of the anecdotal record
4. practice with simulated patient scenarios

Development of a Patient Condition Profile. When gathering information about the patient in preparing for the first appointment

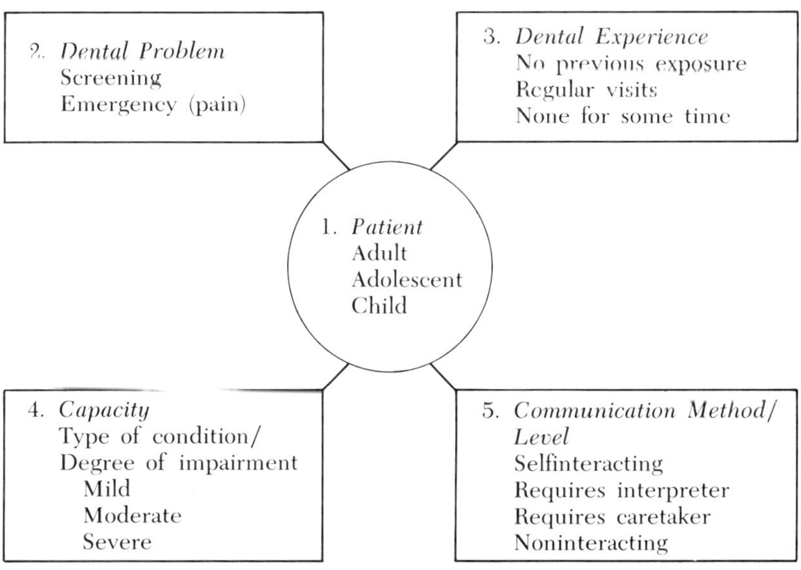

Fig. 1–1. Preparing for the first appointment.

(Fig. 1–1), the following data will allow you to establish a base for problem assessment:

1. the patient's age
2. the dental problem
3. the patient's dental experience
4. the patient's handicapping condition, degree of impairment, and the patient's capacity for interaction
5. the patient's method and level of communication

Acquisition of the additional information presented in Table 1–2 by telephone or during the initial interview will enable the dental team to better plan for the first and subsequent appointments. Consultation with the patient's physicians and other professionals involved may also provide valuable data or assistance with financial, transportation, or home care problems.

Application of a Problem-Solving Assessment Technique. Decisions about handling patient problems can be reached through a systematic pattern of evaluating the problem parameters and determining

TABLE 1–2. Information to be Obtained Prior to First Appointment.

- I. Description of the Handicapping Condition
  - A. Type
  - B. Age at onset
  - C. Name, phone number of physician(s) and other professionals
- II. Patient's Health Status
  - A. Degree of muscle and/or bone involvement
    1. Sites
    2. Stage of involvement
    3. Degree of impaired function
  - B. Treatment regimens
    1. Medications
    2. Therapy schedules
    3. Braces/splints, surgery
    4. Special diets
    5. Adaptive aids
  - C. Emotional status
  - D. Educational/vocational programs
  - E. Special needs, e.g., wheelchair transfers
- III. Dental Status
  - A. History of dental problems
  - B. Past professional care
  - C. Current home care procedures
  - D. Parental/other professional dental concerns
  - E. Dietary pattern(s)
  - F. Attitudes of patient/parent toward dental care
- IV. Prognosis for Dental Management
  - A. Importance of esthetics versus function
  - B. Projected living arrangements/mobility during advanced stages of condition
  - C. Responsibilities for oral hygiene care

alternative approaches for management. The systematic pattern includes:

1. identifying the problem
2. collecting the relevant information or data
3. assessing the problem parameters
4. anticipating the patient's need(s)
5. determining approaches to solving the problem
6. evaluating the results (successful, unresolved, change, discuss)

Table 1–3 (taken from a patient scenario in Chapter 2) demonstrates the application of the systematic pattern of problem solving.

Use of the Anecdotal Record. The anecdotal record is simply a note of any significant fact that will help you maintain effective, positive interaction with the patient or improve a negative interaction. These notes can easily be kept on 3 × 5 or 4 × 6 cards in the patient's record and should be available for all staff members to use or review before subsequent visits. Two different colored cards or pens can be used to distinguish positive versus negative behaviors and actions.

The anecdotal records become important when developing the problem-solving techniques previously described. They can include statements made by the patient or caretaker, or observations or perceptions made by any member of the dental team. Notes should also include changes in approach that proved to be effective or personalization of standard treatment plans for a particular patient. Approaches that are successful with one patient may not be successful with another who has the same handicapping condition.

PRACTICE WITH SIMULATED PATIENT SCENARIOS

The patient scenarios at the end of each chapter are designed to trigger discussions in applying the concepts of normalization and in developing skills in applying the problem-solving assessment technique. There are no right or wrong answers. The scenarios are intended to sharpen your awareness in analyzing patient problems and needs.

Each scenario consists of a brief description of the patient or problem, some of the anticipated patient needs, and a set of questions that form the nucleus of awareness strategies related to the handicapping condition. The anticipated needs and questions are by no means self-limiting. As you become familiar with each condition, you will undoubtedly be able to identify additional needs and questions about each simulated patient.

TABLE 1–3. Systematic Pattern of Problem Solving

1. Patient Concern	2. Data	3. Assessment	4. Need	5. Approach	6. Result
Child has fallen, injuring tooth	3 years old—screaming and crying. Parents are patients.	New environment for child; may be in pain or fearful or both. Parents are familiar with office staff.	Requires soothing and calming, exam and x-ray	• let mother hold child • use mother as interpreter • use mother as model • speak in a warm, soft voice • be patient • reward quickly • show pictures • hold hands with child • use mirror after treatment • give instructions to mother	

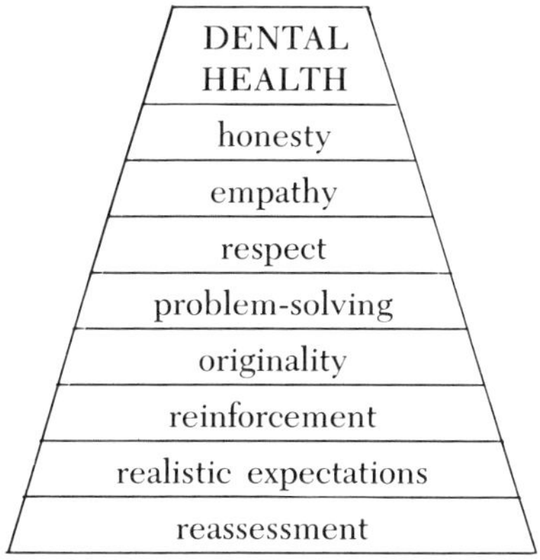

Fig. 1–2. Keys to successful preventive programs.

The preventive aspects and approaches described in each chapter are based on the identification of risk factors that may increase a handicapped individual's susceptibility to dental disease. The goals of this approach are (1) to maximize positive health behaviors, (2) to eliminate risk factors, and (3) to eliminate existing disease.[10] The oral health needs of handicapped people living and working in the community are widely varied; thus, the need for preventive dental health programs for the handicapped has expanded over the last few years to include individuals participating in community-based programs. Many individuals are multiply handicapped and need individualized preventive programs. Knowledge of the medical, psychosocial, and dental implications of the various handicapping conditions, combined with the keys to success identified in Figure 1–2, will permit the dental hygienist and dental assistant to contribute to comprehensive dental care appropriate for the individual needs of each handicapped person and to develop new and better ways to meet the oral health needs of the handicapped.

REFERENCES

1. Federal Register, Vol. 42, No. 86, Wednesday, May 4, 1977. Department of Health, Education and Welfare, p. 22678.
2. Nirje, B.: The normalization principle and its human management implications. *In* Changing Patterns in Residential Services for the Mentally Retarded. Edited by R. Kigel and W. Wolfensberger. Washington, D.C., President's Committee on Mental Retardation, 1969.
3. Wolfensberger, W.: The Principle of Normalization in Human Services. Toronto, National Institute for Mental Retardation, 1972.
4. Ingalls, R.P.: Mental Retardation: The Changing Outlook. New York, John Wiley and Sons, 1978.
5. Neisworth, J.T., and Smith, R.: Retardation: Issues and Assessments and Intervention. New York, McGraw Hill, 1978.
6. Biehl, G.: Guide to the Section 504 Self-Evaluation for Colleges and Universi-

ties. Washington, D.C., National Association of College and University Business Offices, 1978.
7. Special Report: Dental Care for Handicapped Americans. Princeton, N.J., Robert Wood Johnson Foundation, 1979.
8. Program Summaries, National Conference on Dental Care for Handicapped Americans. J. Dent. Educ., *44*(3):154–157, March, 1980.
9. Watson, S., and Tupper, C.: Role of auxiliaries in dental care. *In* Dental Public Health and Community Dentistry. Edited by A. Jong. St. Louis, C.V. Mosby, 1981.
10. Casamassimo, P.S., and Entwistle, B.A.: Prevention for the person with a disability. *In* Dentistry for the Handicapped. Edited by M.M. Album. New York, Masson Publishing (In Press).

Chapter

2 HEARING IMPAIRMENT

Individuals with hearing impairments face a number of problems unique to this handicapping condition. Ironically, perhaps the most significant and socially devastating problem arises from their normal appearance. Hearing-impaired persons are usually not distinguishable from others around them—until communication is attempted. The expectation created by their normal appearance does not prepare others for a lack of response, manual communication, or monotone sounding speech. Without the capacity to understand speech, the hearing impaired are kept from sharing feelings, understanding, appreciation, hopes, and values that are normally conveyed through language.[1,2] It is important for all members of the dental health team to understand the causes of and problems related to hearing impairment in order to plan and conduct a rewarding dental experience for the patient.

DEFINITION AND INCIDENCE

"Hearing impairment" is a term used to describe difficulty in hearing. The term implies defective but functional hearing. A person is considered deaf when she or he is unable to understand speech even with the use of a hearing aid.

The number of people considered deaf or hard of hearing varies, depending upon the definitions used and the source of the data. Conservative estimates indicate approximately nine million people have some type of hearing impairment. Of these people, 8.5 million have hearing losses that create a mild inconvenience or slight handicap. Another 350,000 are auditorily handicapped to a significant degree and require special attention for their hearing loss. Approximately 40,000 of these attend schools for the deaf.

Hearing losses have been noted to accompany a number of other handicapping conditions. Ninety percent of cleft palate patients experience periodic hearing loss from recurrent otitis media.[3] Twenty percent of all persons with cerebral palsy exhibit a high frequency loss.[4] Over 70% of individuals with Down's syndrome demonstrate a permanent conductive hearing loss as a result of recurrent otitis media and a rare structural defect of the middle ear.[5] Hearing loss is common in people with craniofacial anomalies if the structures of the ear or the auditory nerve are abnormal.

Technical advances over the last few decades have led to a better understanding of the causes of hearing impairment, the mechanics of sound, expansion of treatment options, and improved educational techniques.

REVIEW OF ANATOMY AND PHYSIOLOGY

A review of the structure and function of the ear may be helpful in understanding the causes of hearing impairment and the function of sound, treatment choices, and other aspects of hearing impairment.

The human ear consists of three major divisions: the external ear, the middle ear, and the internal ear (Fig. 2–1). The cartilaginous structure of the outer ear, the pinna, is of no functional use, but is important for esthetics. The function of the ear canal is to channel sound into the middle ear. The tympanic membrane (ear drum) separates the external ear from the middle ear cavity. The tympanic membrane is airtight. Pressure in the middle ear is equalized by the process of swallowing, which allows air to enter the Eustachian tube. Pressure on both sides of the tympanic membrane must be equal to allow the membrane to vibrate normally. The function of the middle ear is to transmit vibrations of the tympanic membrane to the internal ear.

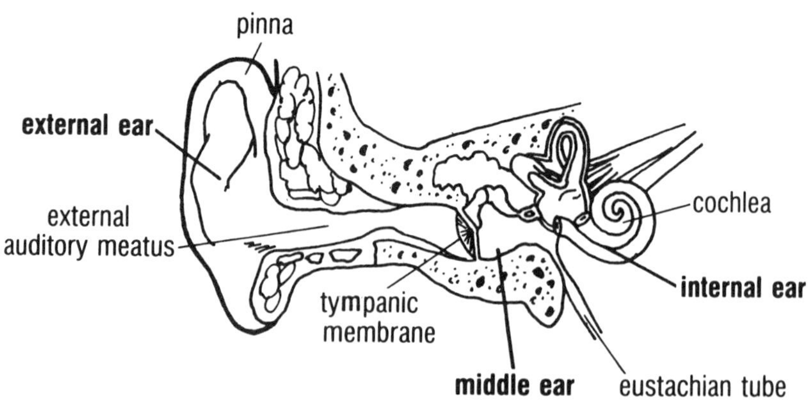

Fig. 2–1. Structure of the human ear.

TABLE 2–1. Hearing Loss and Probable Effects.

Classification	dB Loss	Hearing Without Amplification
Normal range	0–15 dB	All speech sounds
Slight loss	15–25 dB	Hears vowel sounds clearly; may miss unvoiced consonant sounds
Mild loss	25–40 dB	Hears only louder voiced speech sounds
Moderate loss	40–65 dB	Misses most speech at normal conversational level
Severe loss	65–95 dB	Misses all speech at normal conversational level
Profound loss	95+ dB	Hears no speech or other sounds

The internal ear contains the shell-like organ of hearing, the cochlea. Vibrations in the liquid-filled canals of the cochlea are converted into nerve impulses by the organ of Corti and are sent to the brain by the auditory nerve.[6,7]

Frequency and Intensity of Sound. Sound is the result of a vibrating body that sends vibrations in all directions. The vibrations have the characteristics of frequency and intensity, both determined by the source. *Frequency* is the length of the sound wave. The frequency, or vibrations per second, is referred to as cycles per second (CPS). The human range for frequencies is 16 CPS to 30,000 CPS. Generally the higher frequencies are best perceived in early childhood, and perception gradually decreases throughout life so that by the time adulthood is reached, the upper end of the audible range is around 12,000 CPS.

The *intensity* of sound is measured in decibels (dB). One decibel is the faintest intensity that can be heard. The uppermost intensity is 100 dB. An ordinary conversation with a speaker three or four feet away measures about 60 dB. Hearing losses are typically reported in loss of intensity (dBs).[6,8,10] Table 2–1 depicts ranges of dB loss with corresponding effects on hearing.

Recent studies suggest that even a slight hearing impairment is more devastating than once thought. Students with hearing losses in the 15 to 25 dB range have been found to score significantly lower than those with losses of less than 15 dB on all language related subtests of the Stanford achievement tests. Even mild (25 to 40 dB) temporary hearing losses due to recurrent and chronic middle ear infections resulted in deficiencies on tests that require the receiving and processing of auditory stimuli or the production of a verbal response. As a result of studies conducted in England, a hearing loss of 20 dB is considered a significant loss or a handicapping condition.[9]

TYPES OF HEARING LOSS

Hearing impairment may be congenital or acquired at any time as a result of infection, injury, the aging process, or prolonged exposure to noise. Types of hearing loss are classified as: (1) congenital conductive, (2) congenital sensorineural, (3) acquired conductive, and (4) acquired sensorineural. Conductive hearing loss occurs as the result of any injury or disease that interferes with the organs that conduct sound waves through the outer or middle ear. In conductive hearing loss, the inner ear is normal. A conductive hearing loss is usually consistent over the entire range of sound. Patients with conductive loss benefit most from the use of hearing aids.

Sensorineural impairment in hearing results from a malfunction of the organs that perceive sound: the inner ear, the auditory nerve, or the auditory center in the brain. The most common cause of sensorineural hearing loss is the aging process. Of the approximately 20 million Americans over age 65, over 6 million have sufficient bilateral hearing loss to be considered impaired.[6,7,10,11]

Sensorineural impairment involves loss of sensitivity and a reduction in acuity that is generally confined to one or more frequencies, usually the higher frequencies. Since consonants have a higher pitch than vowels and are usually pronounced with less intensity than vowels, difficulties arise in understanding speech. This type of hearing loss is permanent.

Not all hearing losses are purely conductive or sensorineural in nature; some people may have a combination of both types. For these people, treatment is complicated because the hearing loss represents the cumulative problems of both conditions.

TREATMENT OF HEARING LOSS

Treatment of a hearing impairment depends on: (1) the patient's age at onset, (2) the type of impairment, and (3) the cause of the impairment. Several disciplines are usually involved in the diagnosis and development of treatment plans for people with hearing impairments. In the case of children who are deaf, a team approach is employed to ensure optimal development of communication skills. Treatment may include surgery, use of hearing aids, or education geared to the development of communication skills. Educational programs attempt to capitalize on hearing-impaired children's normal curiosity in exploring new environments and their ability to respond to symbols.[2,12,13]

TABLE 2–2. Types of Hearing Aids.

Type of Aid	Characteristics	Indications for Use
Body type hearing aid (monoaural or binaural)	Most powerful and durable, least cosmetic, broad frequency range	Used primarily for children and people with profound losses in whom power output is more important than cosmetics
Bone-conduction hearing aid	Used in body or eyeglass types; bone oscillator worn with a headband or as part of eyeglass bow	Used for people with a conductive loss that is not surgically correctable
Behind-the-ear aid	Most common; most esthetic; often good localization and isolation of signals	Can be used for the majority of hearing losses
Eyeglass aid	Cosmetic appeal; broad range of frequency responses	Usually for people who wear eyeglasses but object to the behind-the-ear type aid
CROS and BICROS aid	Microphone placed over worst ear; requires only slight amplification	Used for people with precipitous hearing loss
In-the-ear aid	Cosmetic, but much distortion and feedback	Used only for mild losses

A variety of hearing aids are available, depending on the type and severity of the loss and patient preference. Common types are described in Table 2–2. New areas of research include acupuncture treatment for deafness, implantable aids, and direct stimulation of the auditory nerve.[14]

PSYCHOSOCIAL IMPLICATIONS

The effect of a hearing loss on development of communication skills depends on the age at onset, the duration of loss, and the frequency of the fluctuations in hearing. Congenital deafness is a severe disability that drastically alters the development of communication skills.

Children who have hearing impairments may have delayed or impaired language development, be educationally behind their peers, or exhibit a higher frequency of behavioral problems.[2,15,16] Adults who are deaf are generally well adjusted and have learned to compensate. However, biases and prejudices still exist that directly or indirectly affect these individuals. For instance, over 80% of adult males classified as deaf are relegated to manual labor jobs.[9,10]

ORAL MANIFESTATIONS

Specific oral manifestations are not generally associated with hearing impairments unless the hearing loss is a result of a syndrome such as ectodermal dysplasia. People with hearing impairments due to prematurity or rubella may exhibit enamel dysplasia because of the interrupted dental development. Bruxism has also been noted in people with hearing impairments.[16] The severe wear caused by this habit can influence dental treatment planning.

DENTAL MANAGEMENT

When the dental office is contacted by the patient, parent, friend, or agency representative and an appointment is scheduled, the receptionist should determine the following information about the patient's hearing loss:

1. the type of hearing loss
2. the severity of the loss (in terms of actual function)
3. the age of onset and etiology
4. whether a hearing aid is worn
5. how the person generally communicates
6. how to contact the patient if another person is making the initial contact
7. the patient's previous dental experience

It is important not to assume that patients with previous exposure to a dental environment understand what is happening. Alternative methods of communicating effectively must be established. Many adult patients who are deaf may be capable of reading lips. Some individuals are reluctant to divulge this information because of the time it takes to adapt to the various facial expressions and gestures that accompany speaking styles. Lip reading is extremely difficult, particularly if the lips are covered by a moustache or beard. At best, it is only 26% efficient.[3,17]

Other forms of communication such as use of pictures, hand signs, or written messages are available for persons who cannot read lips or benefit from hearing aids. Some patients may be accompanied by a person who can interpret or assist with communication. As the patient gains confidence, the interpreter should take a less active role.

Sign language is the most common form of communication among people in the U.S. who are deaf. Signing is often supplemented by finger spelling. You may want to learn and practice a few signs that will help put your patient at ease[18] (Fig. 2–2). Signing should always be accompanied by spoken language. Mueller and Gantl provide an excellent overview of some helpful signs.[17]

Prior to the appointment, the dental team members may write information on cards for the patient, especially if the anticipated treatment is complicated and the patient's hearing is severely compromised. This could take the form of (1) a step-by-step sequence of the anticipated examination and treatment, (2) identification of staff, and (3) expectations for treatment. The liberal use of drawings and pictures with a minimum of written messages will help facilitate communication with children.

If the patient plans to be accompanied by an interpreter or parent, a member of the dental staff should explain to the person in advance what will transpire in the dental office.[19] This person should be encouraged to stress the positive aspects in preparing the patient for the visit.

Meeting the Patient. When meeting the patient, face him or her when you speak so your lip movements and facial expressions can be observed. Pronounce words carefully and distinctly. People often make the mistake of yelling or talking very slowly. Conversation should be conducted at a normal rate and tone. If the patient cannot understand you, restate your instructions or explanation in dif-

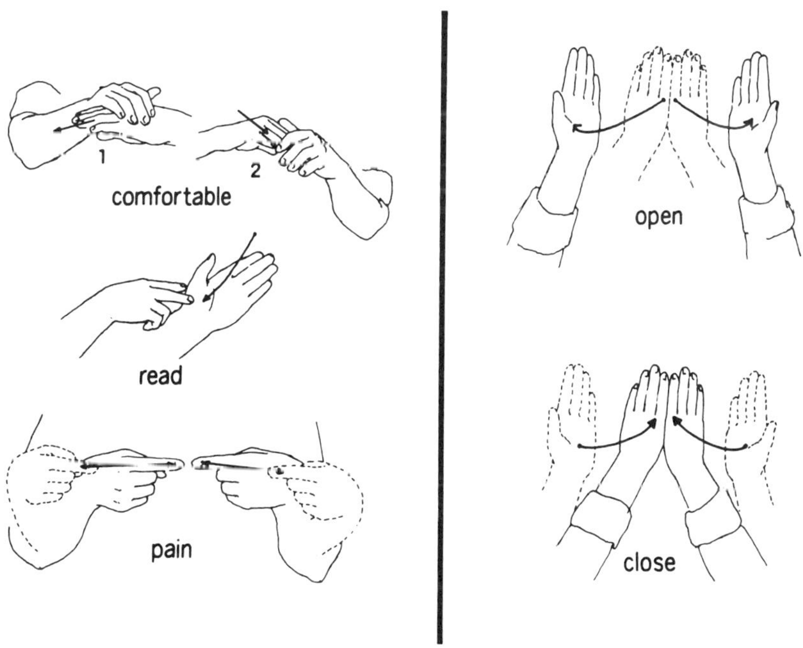

Fig. 2–2. Selected concept hand signs.

ferent words, since some words are harder for the patient to read than others. Avoid dropping your voice at the end of a sentence. This is the time when the patient's perception of the dental environment will begin to take shape, so gentle facial expressions, warm tone of voice, and calm, efficient manner are important. You need to convey a respect for the individual, whether child or adult, and not indicate frustration with the situation or a fear of the patient's behavior. If your patient attempts to speak, try to understand what she or he is saying. If you cannot understand what is being said, suggest a written message. Have paper and pencil ready.

If the patient is a child, have the parent bring him or her early and spend some time showing them around the office while observing their mood, method of communicating with each other, and the tone established between them. The parent may be fearful or enthusiastic; the child, overly dependent or calm and responsive. Holding a child's hand, letting him touch things, and making sure he can see you at all times are ways of building rapport.

When explaining procedures to the patient, you may want to have written words, pictures, models, and actual instruments to use for step-by-step demonstration, drawing attention to the relationship of the words and pictures to the models and the objects. This is also a good time to use the concept symbols you may have learned, to establish responses from the patient for "pain," "start," "stop," "open," "bite down," and other key words. Question the patient at the midpoint and the end of your explanation to determine if she or he understands what is going to happen. Head-nodding and smiling by the patient may be an expression of encouragement or nervousness and not an expression of understanding.

Anecdotal notes of any significant facts that will help you to maintain an effective interaction should be written in the dental record. Simple notes are sufficient: "Charles is always called 'Bud,'" or "Mr. Smith reads lips very well—has no problem understanding," or "Bobby cried until we let him try out the dental chair." As described in Chapter 1, these anecdotes are important for future visits and for communication among members of the staff. They also serve to individualize each patient's record, for not all hearing-impaired patients will present the same problems.[15,19]

DENTAL TREATMENT

Once treatment begins, remember that the patient cannot use the auditory sense as a cue to the presence of those around him. The patient will be startled if you attempt to touch without main-

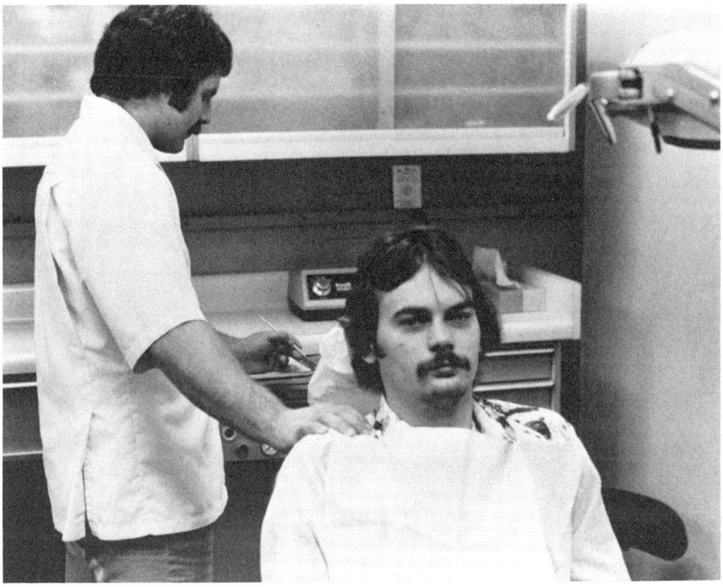

Fig. 2–3. Maintaining of physical contact is necessary to avoid startling a deaf patient.

taining physical or visual contact[20] (Fig. 2–3).

As each step in the treatment is introduced, explanation and demonstration are indicated. Any change of equipment should take place directly in front of the patient. The lip-reading patient will have a difficult time unless you are sure not to interrupt the line of vision with your hands or with instruments. Hearing-impaired persons are particularly sensitive to vibrations, so be sure to identify the introduction of high-speed handpieces and ultrasonic scalers. Hearing aids may be turned down or removed for maximum comfort, and reset or replaced as soon as possible. "O" indicates off; "M" means microphone (on). Consultation with the patient or caretaker will assist you in learning about the different types of aids and determining patient preference for the volume settings during treatment.

Include the patient's tactile and visual senses in your demonstrations, particularly with children. The fingernail can be used to demonstrate such steps as the vibration of the polisher, the feeling of the scaler, and the flow of the air syringe. Demonstrating on models, showing the child x-rays, and showing the teeth in the mirror are all ways of keeping the child stimulated and involved (Fig. 2–4). A careful explanation is required in preparing the patient for the administration of anesthesia and the resulting feeling that he or she will experience.[3]

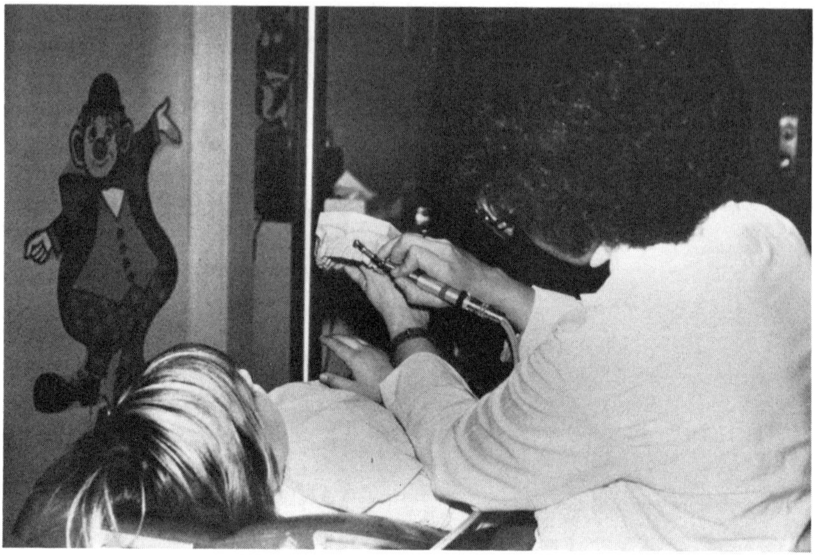

Fig. 2–4. Maintaining children's interest through stimulation helps to reduce anxiety.

PREVENTIVE MEASURES

For adults, home care instructions ideally should consist of instructional material written on cards, demonstrated on a model, and then demonstrated in the patient's mouth. This middle step can often be omitted if you think intraoral instruction with observation in a mirror is the most effective method. This should be followed by a demonstration of the patient's understanding of what is being taught to facilitate correction or modification of any errors. The educational sequence should be the same for children, but pictures or drawings may have to be substituted for written cards. When possible, the person responsible for the child's care should be present throughout the educational sequence and their role in home care clarified. Many adults and children with hearing impairments can benefit from the use of disclosing solution as a means of identifying plaque and areas missed in brushing. Patients should be encouraged to use the disclosing procedure as a means of self-monitoring their oral hygiene.

FOLLOW-UP

Appointment reminders or appointment changes can be made through the mail or with a parent or friend, or by calling the number of a person willing to take a message. Following the appointment, all members of the team should review the visit (1) to identify the strengths and weaknesses of the appointment sequence, (2) to complete the anecdotal notes, and (3) to make notes in the record about considerations for the next appointment.

If the child is receiving special services in school and toothbrushing is incorporated into the program, consultation with the teacher or therapists about oral hygiene care may prove beneficial. Such communication will provide a chance to discuss the oral care recommendations that were given at the dental office and to exchange ideas about providing effective dental health education.

PATIENT SCENARIOS

Patient 1

Description

Three-year-old Cindy has just fallen and injured one of her teeth. Cindy has been deaf from birth. Her mother and father are regular patients. An emergency appointment is made for Cindy. This is her first visit to the dentist. She arrives screaming and crying.

Anticipated Needs

—an examination to determine extent of injury and pain
—x-rays
—treatment if necessary

Awareness Strategies

1. How will you communicate with Cindy? How can you differentiate whether she's in pain or just frightened?
2. What role should the parents play during the appointment?
3. How will you prepare Cindy for the examination and subsequent procedures, particularly the x-ray?

Patient 2

Description

Your office has just received a call from Mrs. Samson, who is new in town and was referred to your office by a neighbor. She does not know the area at all. She is 68 years old and has recently been fitted with new dentures, which are bothering her. Her former dentist treated her for 30 years. She has a moderate to severe acquired hearing loss and wears a hearing aid.

Anticipated Needs

—home care instructions
—nutritional instructions

—assurances about her dental status
—dental adjustment by the dentist
—follow-up appointment

Awareness Strategies

1. How can you determine the severity of Mrs. Samson's hearing loss? What information should you gather over the telephone?
2. How can you allay her anxieties?
3. How might you give home care instructions?
4. Should you remove her hearing aid during treatment?

Patient 3

Description

Mary is 26 years old and has been completely deaf since age 13, following a serious illness. She still has residual medical problems. She reads lips and uses sign language fluently. She requires a comprehensive examination, as she has not seen a dentist in several years.

Anticipated Needs

—complete prophylaxis
—x-rays
—extensive treatment plan
—home care instructions

Awareness Strategies

1. What information should you acquire over the phone?
2. What signs might be useful in communicating with Mary?
3. What other techniques might aid in explaining treatment procedures to her?
4. How can you make Mary feel at ease?

REFERENCES

1. Meadow, K.P., and Trybus, R.J.: Behavioral and emotional problems of deaf children: An overview. *In* Hearing and Hearing Impairment. Edited by L.J. Bradford and W.G. Hardy. New York, Grune & Stratton, 1979.
2. Kates, S.L.: Language Development in Deaf and Hearing Adolescents. Northampton, Mass., Dept. of Health, Education and Welfare, 1972.
3. Tunes, W., and Dexter, C.: Dentistry and the hearing impaired child. J. Pedodont., *3*(4):321–334, 1979.
4. Nober, E.H.: Auditory processing. *In* Cerebral Palsy: A Developmental Disability, 3rd ed. Edited by W.C. Cruickshank. Syracuse, Syracuse University Press, 1976.
5. Northein, J.L., and Davis, M. (eds.): Communicative disorders in Down's syndrome. Seminars in Speech, Language and Hearing, *1*(1):1–97, 1980.

6. Gulick, L.W.: Hearing: Physiology and Psychophysics. New York, Oxford University Press, 1971.
7. Snow, J.B. Physiology of hearing. *In* Hearing Loss in Children: A Comprehensive Text. Edited by B.E. Jaffe. Baltimore, University Park Press, 1977.
8. Hughes, L.F., and Berlin, C.I.: Physics of sound and the decibel. *In* Hearing Disorders. Edited by J. Northern. Boston, Little, Brown, 1976.
9. Binne, C.A.: Relevant aural rehabilitation. *In* Hearing Disorders. Editd by J. Northern. Boston, Little, Brown, 1976.
10. Downs, M.P.: The handicap of deafness. *In* Hearing Disorders. Edited by J. Northern. Boston, Little, Brown, 1976.
11. Beadle, K.R.: Communication disorders—speech and hearing. *In* Physically Handicapped Children. Edited by E.E. Bleck and D.A. Nagel. New York, Grune & Stratton, 1975.
12. Schwab, W.A.: Effects of hearing loss on education. *In* Hearing Loss in Children: A Comprehensive Text. Edited by B.E. Jaffe. Baltimore, University Park Press, 1977.
13. Stidwell, M.: John Tracy Clinic Language Guide. Los Angeles, The John Tracy Clinic, 1976.
14. Northern, J.L. (ed.): Hearing Disorders. Boston, Little, Brown, 1976.
15. Stewart, J.M.: Medical management of the hearing handicapped child. *In* Hearing Disorders. Edited by J. Northern. Boston, Little, Brown, 1976.
16. Kanar, H.L.: The blind and the deaf. *In* Dentistry for the Handicapped. Edited by H.J. Nowak. St. Louis, C.V. Mosby, 1976.
17. Mueller, K., and Gantl, D.: Communicating with the deaf patient. J. Dent. for Handicapped, *3*(2):22–25, 1978.
18. O'Rourke, T.J.: A Basic Course in Manual Communication. 2nd ed. Silver Springs, Md., National Association of the Deaf, 1974.
19. Brownstein, M.P.: Dental care for the deaf child. *In* Dent. Clin. North Am., *18*(3):643–650, 1974.
20. Wilkins, E.M.: Clinical Practice of the Dental Hygienist. 4th ed. Philadelphia, Lea & Febiger, 1976.

Chapter 3

VISUAL IMPAIRMENTS AND BLINDNESS

What are your feelings when you meet or observe a person who is blind? Concern? Pity? Amazement they can maneuver by themselves? Have you ever wondered whether you should offer assistance? Many people do not know how to respond to such situations or know enough about blindness or visual impairment to be comfortable. As a result, the true abilities and talents of blind and visually impaired persons often are underestimated. An understanding of the abilities and limitations of those suffering from this handicap will help to facilitate the provision of quality dental care.

DEFINITION

A person who has received the best optical correction and can see at 20 feet in the best eye what a person with normal vision can see at 200 feet is considered legally blind (visual acuity of 20/200 or less) (Fig. 3–1). A person is also considered legally blind if the corrected field of vision is less than an angle of 20°.[1] A person is considered visually impaired if, after the best optical correction, the visual acuity in the best eye is no better than 20/70. The definition of visual impairment is not limited to overall corrected sight of 20/70; it also includes visual limitations due to the loss of peripheral or central vision (Fig. 3–2). Most individuals meeting the foregoing definitions are eligible for orientation and adjustment, educational and vocational rehabilitation training services offered by various community agencies.

INCIDENCE

The National Society for the Prevention of Blindness and agencies that provide services to persons who are blind estimate that about 450,000 Americans are legally blind. Approximately half of

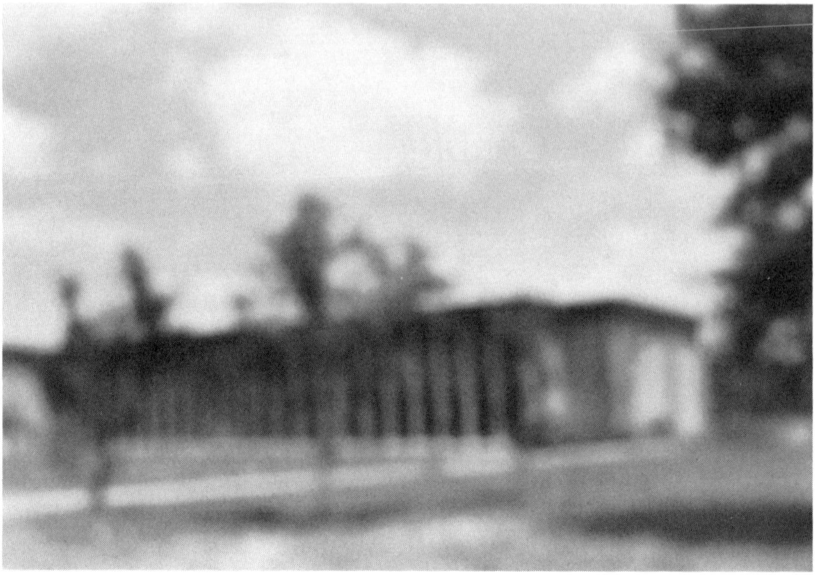

Fig. 3–1. Visual acuity of approximately 20/200.

these individuals are 60 years of age or older; 10% are school age or younger.[1] Data suggest, however, that about 25% of all school age children have visual impairments, the majority of which are correctable if treatment were provided.[2] Because of the changing pattern in the prevalence of blindness, the majority of visually impaired persons today have additional handicaps.

ETIOLOGY

The major causes of blindness include trauma, disease (infections, inflammation, or toxicity), and structural or developmental defects. During the last 40 years, the incidence of blindness as a result of injury has decreased markedly and currently accounts for less than 3% of reported cases. Requirements for safety glasses in certain occupational settings and careful monitoring of fireworks and potentially dangerous toys have contributed to the decrease. Blindness due to certain diseases, such as infections at birth, congenital syphilis, and trachoma, has also declined in certain parts of the world. The relationship between retrolental fibroplasia and blindness was discovered in the 1950s and measures were instituted to alleviate the problem. Retrolental fibroplasia occurs when premature infants are placed in incubators containing a high concentration of oxygen. The excess oxygen causes hemorrhage of the retinal blood vessels, eventually leading to formation of fibrotic scar tissue, retinal detachment, and blindness. Unfortunately, this condition still occurs needlessly.

Antibiotic usage significantly decreased the incidence of disease-

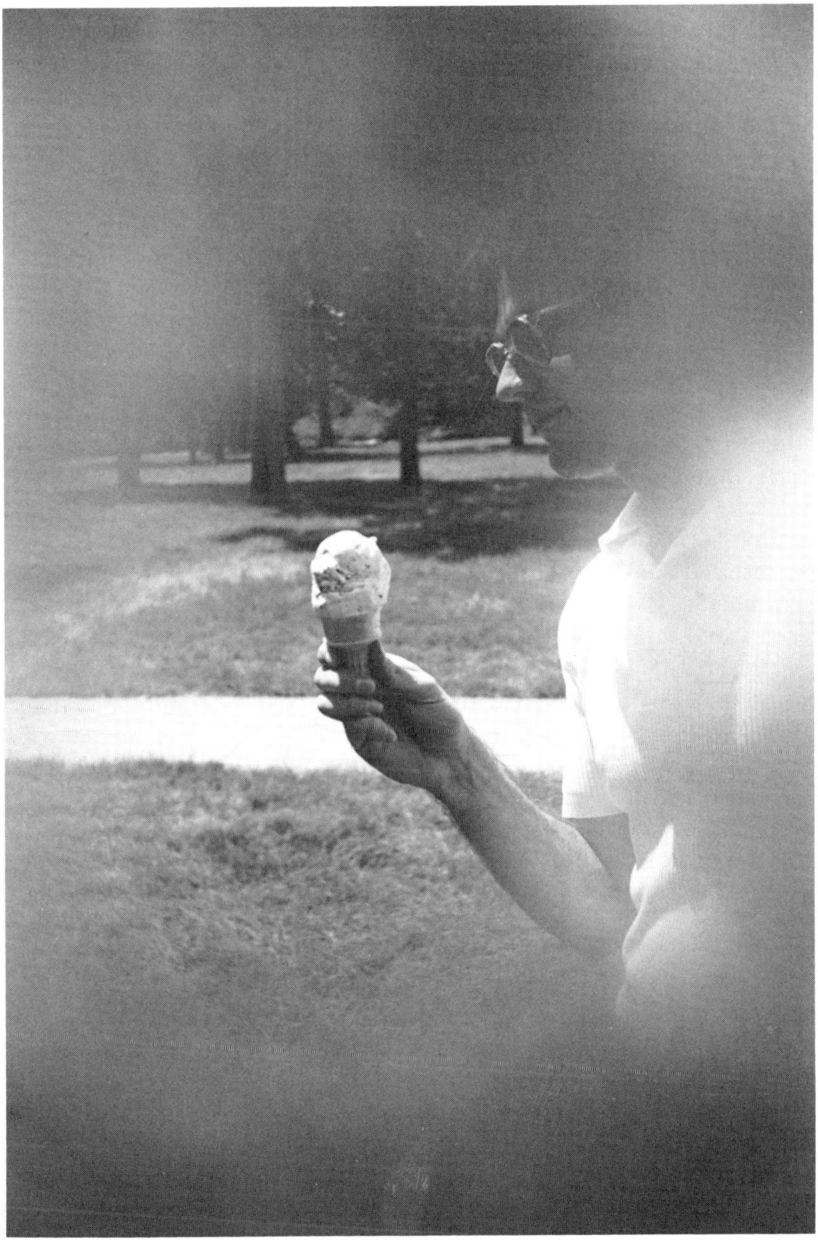

Fig. 3–2. Loss of peripheral vision.

induced blindness. Viruses such as the rubella virus (German measles), however, have continued to infect pregnant females in the first trimester to cause multiple congenital abnormalities, such as congenital cataracts, heart defects, and hearing loss.

Blindness or visual impairments may be one of several physical or other abnormalities associated with genetic disorders or other prenatal insults. Examples of these anomalies include lens dislocation, strabismus, and optic nerve defects. These anomalies often are seen as a component of a syndrome.[3]

Currently, macula degeneration (loss of central vision), complications of diabetes (retinal hemorrhages), glaucoma (failure of the liquid in the eye to drain, causing pressure, pain, and blindness), and cataracts (clouding of the lens, thus blocking light perception) are among the leading causes of blindness in the United States.[4,5,6]

TREATMENT

Early diagnosis of eye disorders often improves prognosis by limiting the extent of damage to the eye. Early diagnosis also permits early initiation of treatment and education. Regular eye examinations by an ophthalmologist (including tests for glaucoma and amblyopia), the use of safety glasses in areas where eye injury can occur, and immediate medical attention for obvious or suspected eye injury or infection are the cornerstones of preventing unnecessary eye impairments.

The goal of intervention and treatment is to improve sight and to prevent further impairment of vision. The treatment of choice varies with the type and severity of impairment.[7] Surgery for cataracts is reportedly effective in 95% of the cases. Treatment for glaucoma entails reducing the intraocular pressure through drugs, surgery, or both. Research is ongoing to discover new drugs and the use of laser beams to improve the prognosis of certain disorders of the eye.

EDUCATIONAL PROGRAMS

Educational programs for blind and visually impaired persons are determined to some extent by their age at onset of the disability. Children who are congenitally blind learn very differently from children or adults who become adventitiously blind. Most programs teach reliance on auditory instruction, memory, and more effective use of the tactile or other senses. Auditory instruction includes the use of talking books, audio cassette tapes, voice-guided direction, and instruction in educating others to give effective verbal information. Training in the tactile sense includes the use of Braille (a system of raised dots) for reading, writing, and typing. Braille is currently used by about 10% of the blind population. Persons with some degree of visual impairment have benefited from large-print books and other low-vision aids. Valuable research is continuing in the application of computer technology to reading machines.

Educational programs also include instruction in independent living skills, such as clothing care (especially color coordination), preparation of meals, housecleaning, and travel. Travel is facilitated by clear path indicators, long canes, and dog guides. One-fare travel concessions also permit a legally blind person and a companion to travel together for a single fare. Education of blind and visually impaired individuals is no longer confined to private schools or colleges or segregated special education classes. In 1972, over 60% of blind children in this country attended public or private day schools.[1] These students are mainstreamed into regular classrooms and receive services through resource rooms and itinerant teachers.

PSYCHOSOCIAL IMPLICATIONS

Assuming that blindness or visual impairment is not combined with other disabilities, the blind or visually impaired individual is fully capable of becoming an independent, productive member of society. The major problems encountered by blind and visually impaired persons are the attitudes and behavior of uninformed members of society, reflected in such daily occurrences as: (1) unsolicited and inappropriate assistance by strangers; (2) people talking in a loud voice as if the person were deaf; (3) addressing questions to sighted companions; or (4) verbalizing pity. Blind and visually impaired individuals are subjected to these injustices by a society that does not expect them to be competent and does not realize that blindness can be reduced to the level of a physical nuisance if proper training opportunities and daily application of skills are available.[8]

For those with congenital blindness, the provision of appropriate learning opportunities to facilitate independent living should begin in childhood. Parents and caretakers need to cope with their feelings of guilt, confusion, injustice, and anger about conceiving or raising a blind or visually impaired child. Once the parents or caretakers begin to work through their feelings, they can proceed with structuring a home environment that is stimulating and challenging, yet supportive. Stimulation includes the freedom to explore one's environment without being unduly confined to avoid accidents. Parental overprotection and restriction generally results in an overly dependent child who manifests a number of behavioral and emotional problems. In addition, stereotypic and self-stimulatory behavior, such as rocking and eye-poking, are nonproductive and should be discouraged because they impede learning of socially appropriate behaviors and other activities.[9]

ORAL MANIFESTATIONS

Unless a blind or visually impaired person has one or more disabilities in addition to his visual disorder, oral abnormalities can be expected to occur at the same rate as in the sighted population.[6] However, the rate of periodontal disease may be higher if oral hygiene is inadequate.[10] Although not documented through research, trauma to the teeth may be more prevalent if the patient trips, falls, or bumps into objects frequently.[11]

DENTAL MANAGEMENT

Dental management considerations depend upon:

1. degree of visual impairment
2. age of onset of visual disability
3. presence of other handicapping conditions
4. degree of independence
5. patient attitude and behavior
6. parental attitude and behavior (if patient is a child or severely handicapped)

When seeking access to dental care, persons with visual impairments may encounter several potential barriers. Choosing a dentist is sometimes complicated by inability to read the yellow pages of the phone book, locate transportation, pay for care, or get release time from work. Persons who use guide dogs can experience problems in relation to negative attitudes about transporting the dog or allowing it to stay in the dental office. Since the majority of visually impaired persons are elderly, multiply handicapped, or medically compromised, various physical aspects of the dental office may prove to be barriers. Long flights of steps, poorly lighted halls, loose rugs, directions listed in small print, unwieldy doors, slippery floors, and sudden changes in surface texture may all prove hazardous to the visually impaired or blind person. Many of these problems can be eliminated by providing directions to and a description of the office, elimination of potential physical barriers in the office, and discussion among the dental staff regarding issues such as guide dogs. Patient information that is generally acquired by written questionnaire can be handled by telling the patient what information is needed for the first appointment and scheduling additional time during the first appointment for a verbal interview.

The blind or visually impaired child, like all children, could benefit from visiting the dental office prior to an appointment. Arrangements can be made for the child to be accompanied by an older sighted sibling, friend, or parent. The visit should consist of becoming familiar with the people, sounds, textures, and smells of the dental office. Preappointment visits can help to desensitize the child and minimize anxious behavior due to unfamiliarity with the people and the environment. Introduction of oral hygiene procedures and parental counseling can also begin at this appointment.[12] Parents should be encouraged to practice looking in the child's mouth to accustom the child to oral examination and dental routines.

Since blind or visually impaired persons have the same wide range of interests, skills, and needs as other persons, no single treatment approach is applicable to all patients. Rather than assuming that the patient has certain needs and skills, the most effective and appreciated approach to patient management is to ASK THE PATIENT what methods he or she prefers. This approach indicates that you are aware of the various options available, yet enables the patient to determine which procedures are easiest and most comfortable for him or her.

Meeting the Patient. As patients are greeted in the waiting room by the receptionist, dental assistant, or dental hygienist, the patient should be acclimated to the layout of the waiting room, introduced to the office dental staff, and informed of the location of coat racks, restrooms, available chairs, and other furniture. When conducting the patient to the operatory or any other room, verbal instructions indicating directions, changes in floor textures, or potential obstacles such as large plants should be given. Physical assistance is often appropriate even if the person uses a cane. Such assistance is best provided by standing slightly in front of the patient and allowing him or her to hold onto a bent arm, usually near the elbow (Fig. 3–3). This allows the patient to be slowly guided (not dragged) through the office. If the person uses a guide dog, both should follow you into the operatory, and the dog allowed to sit in another room after the patient is seated comfortably. Seating is accomplished by guiding the person's hand over the back, arm, and seat portion of the chair, and then allowing him to seat himself. All obstacles such as tray tables, operator chairs, or lights should be removed from the area prior to the patient's being seated. Parents of visually impaired or blind children may be asked to remain in the operatory for the first few sessions to assist with communication and relieve anxiety.

After the patient is seated, he or she should be introduced to other staff members or patients in the operatory, so that people can be recognized by their voices whenever they speak. This will prevent future confusion if more than one person is conversing in the room. To avoid such confusion, one staff member should con-

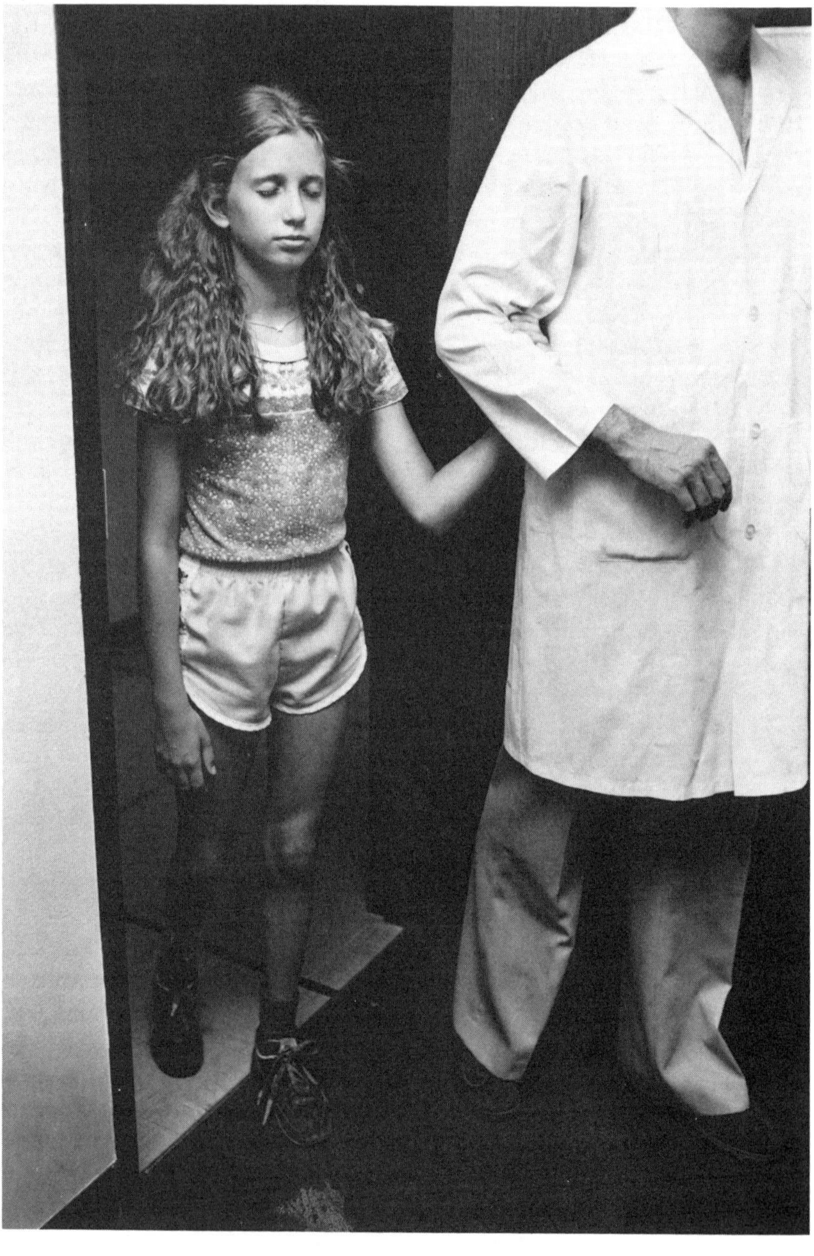

Fig. 3–3. Guided assistance of a patient into a dental office.

duct most of the conversation, with other members identifying themselves occasionally until the patient can comfortably identify each person by the voice. Excess noise such as loud music, prolonged suction, ultrasonic cleaners, or other distractions should be minimized, since the patient cannot visually discriminate which noises are relevant to the particular moment.

DENTAL TREATMENT

Once the patient is seated, the motorized noises and movements of the chair and each piece of equipment should be identified. This can be accomplished by allowing the patient to feel the object while its function is explained. The light sensitivity of visually impaired patients should be determined prior to turning on the dental light, since some individuals are sensitive to bright light. As treatment begins, repeat the explanation about each instrument before placing it in the patient's mouth. Inform the patient as you approach his or her mouth, as tactile stimulation without prior warning may trigger the patient's startle reflex. In a similar manner, smells and tastes unique to the dental environment, such as cavity varnish, prophy paste, or fluoride should be described prior to introduction into the mouth. After the patient becomes familiar with the sounds, smells, and tastes, verbal guidance may be all that is required. Verbal reassurance about the patient's progress will have to substitute in many instances for smiles and body language. Any procedure or occurrence that necessitates the staff member's moving away from the patient, such as procuring an instrument or going to the sink, should be preceded by an explanation of where the person is going so that the patient will not be left talking to an empty chair! In essence, the dental team member must maintain a running conversation that vividly paints a mental picture of the appointment for the patient.

Expectations of the patient's behavior should be outlined at the beginning of the appointment so that the patient understands the forthcoming procedures and how he or she might assist to facilitate treatment or communicate his or her needs and concerns. The use of the suction or cuspidor should be described and the patient informed about which procedures require that his or her head and body remain relatively stable. Providing frequent physical reassurance and stability will create a more comfortable spatial orientation and feeling of security for the patient while reinforcing the image of you as a person. The following dialogue provides an example of how some of these suggestions can be integrated into one portion of an initial dental appointment:

Hygienist: John, I'm going to recline the chair to a position that is comfortable for you and allows me to see inside your mouth better.

John: OK. What makes the chair recline?

Hygienist: (Putting hand on his arm.) As I tilt the chair back now, you'll hear a noise which is the motor that controls the chair.

John: Yes, I hear it. Whoa, I feel as though I'm slipping down in the chair!

Hygienist: (Hand still on arm.) Don't worry, that's as far back as it will tilt. Now you can move up and make yourself comfortable. (Adjusting headrest.) Is that better?

John: Yes, thanks. Now what?

Hygienist: I'm going to turn on a light that makes it easier for me to see everything in your mouth. Does bright light bother you at all?

John: No, I have very little light perception.

Hygienist: (Turning on light.) When I'm examining your teeth, I will need you to open your mouth fairly wide. I don't need it open all the time, however, so I will let you know when I do. I don't want your jaw to become tired.

John: Thanks, my jaw tires very quickly.

Hygienist: Let me know if you're tired or if anything else is a problem. If you need to do this while my hands or instruments are in your mouth, please raise your hand or make some other signal so that I can take my instruments out. If you suddenly move your head or try to talk, my instrument could accidentally slip off your tooth and poke your gum tissue or tongue. That wouldn't feel very good, would it?

John: No, I guess not. What kind of instruments will you be using?

Hygienist: I'll let you feel each one and tell you how I'm going to use it.

PREVENTIVE MEASURES

Dental health education and preventive procedures will probably require certain modifications. Yeadon[13] suggests the use of one-to-one instruction, where the instructor's role is one of tutor and observer. Yeadon's advice should not, however, be interpreted as an endorsement to establish an inflexible step-by-step program of brushing or flossing. Suggestions for home care and preventive pro-

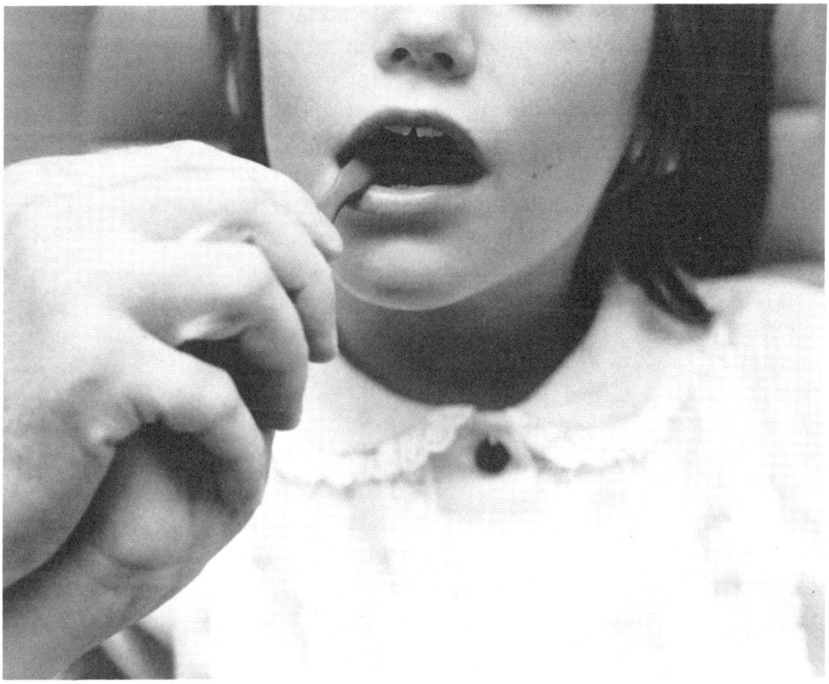

Fig. 3–4. Guided instruction in toothbrushing.

cedures should be offered along with the opportunity for the blind or visually impaired person to adapt the suggestions to his or her skill level. A rigid set of rules or a set way of doing a task can leave the blind or visually impaired person at a loss if the sequence is interrupted or varied.[14]

Instruction in brushing should begin with the patient's demonstrating his or her current brushing technique. Refinements and correction of deficiencies can be accomplished by physical and verbal guidance. Physical guidance consists of placing your hand on the patient's hand and performing brushing together while verbally describing the most appropriate brushing technique (Fig. 3–4). Disclosing solution or tablets can be used to aid in assessing the patient's brushing effectiveness, and should be explained as such. The hygienist or assistant can describe or locate each area of plaque and encourage the patient to brush these areas carefully. Since the patient will not be able to self-monitor effectiveness with this method, he or she should establish a specific sequence of brushing to assure that all areas are brushed adequately. Musical jingles or audiotapes are available to teach such a sequence to children with visual impairments.[15]

Dental health instruction often can be accomplished effectively through the use of self-modeling. Prior to instruction, the patient should wash his or her hands and then be assisted in exploring all structures inside the mouth. The texture of the teeth should be noted before and after brushing. The purpose of brushing (such as good breath and removal of debris) can then be explained and a brushing method demonstrated. Plastic or other models of the mouth have also been used effectively as instructional aids. Lebowitz[16] provides a comprehensive list of teaching materials that may prove helpful with persons who are visually impaired. In addition to models and audiotapes, he includes magnifying aids, large print materials, and raised label markers. These are particularly useful for older individuals who are gradually losing their eyesight. Flossing can be taught in a manner similar to toothbrushing, but may be facilitated by the use of commercially available floss aids. One program taught the concept of flossing by using the patient's fingers to simulate the contour of the interdental papilla.[17] Because of the concentration and emphasis on the tactile sense that they must possess to perform manual procedures, many blind persons master flossing faster than their sighted peers.

The key to successful oral hygiene programs with visually impaired persons involves creating adaptations and routines that allow them to be totally independent in oral hygiene care and to develop pride in their achievements. This includes purchasing oral hygiene materials, labeling or storing materials so that they won't be lost, brushing all areas effectively, and determining whether they have been performing adequately.

PATIENT SCENARIOS

Patient 1

Description

Mrs. Paul calls to set up an appointment for her 16-year-old son, Mark. Mark has been blind since birth and has not had dental care for some time. The family has just moved to the city.

Anticipated Needs

—radiographs
—prophylaxis
—home care instructions

Awareness Strategies

1. How will you interact with a blind teenager in a new environment?

2. Does Mark have any other handicapping conditions to be considered?
3. What encouragement will you give Mark to follow through with home care instructions?
4. How will Mark know what his oral health status is?

Patient 2

Description

Mary Brown is a 36-year-old woman who uses a seeing-eye dog. She knows Braille, is peppy, and works in the library. On her previous visit, one of the patients had complained about the dog in the waiting room.

Anticipated Needs:

—review of home care instructions
—select treatment
—specific radiographs

Awareness Strategies

1. Will you have to review the physical layout with Mary?
2. How will you make Mary comfortable while taking the other patients into consideration?
3. How will you explain the radiographic procedures?
4. How will you help Mary identify areas of improvement in her home care procedures?

Patient 3

Description

The teacher of a preschool for handicapped children has asked you to develop a dental health program for the children. Most of the children have visual and other impairments. She would like you to include oral screenings, oral care instructions, and dental health education. How would you approach the development of the program?

Anticipated Needs

—projected time involvement
—educational materials needed
—equipment requirements
—teaching approaches

Awareness Strategies

1. How will you determine the level of instruction and interaction?

2. Whom can you involve to assist you with individualizing oral care instructions?
3. What kinds of teaching aids should you prepare for these children?
4. Who will be responsible for following up the program?

REFERENCES

1. Dickman, I.R.: Living with Blindness. Public Affairs Pamphlet #473, Public Affairs Comm., 1972.
2. The vision gap. Dental Assistant, *40*:25-26, May, 1971.
3. Fredrickson, D.: Hereditary systemic diseases of metabolism that affect the eye. *In* The Eye and Systemic Disease. Edited by F. Mausolf. St. Louis, C.V. Mosby, 1975.
4. A Step by Step Guide to Personal Management for Blind Persons. New York, American Foundation for the Blind, 1974.
5. Rosenthal, R.: Visual disorders. *In* Physically Handicapped Children: A Medical Atlas for Teachers. Edited by E. Bleck and D. Nagel. New York, Grune & Stratton, 1975.
6. Kanar, H.: The blind and the deaf. *In* Dentistry for the Handicapped Patient. Edited by A. Nowak. St. Louis, C.V. Mosby, 1976.
7. Adams. A., Daniel, A., McCubbin, J., and Rullman, L.: Games, Sports and Exercises for the Physically Handicapped. ed. 2. Philadelphia, Lea & Febiger, 1982.
8. Olson, C.: Blindness can be reduced to an inconvenience. Visual Impairment and Blindness, pp. 406–411, November, 1977.
9. Chapman, E.: Visually Handicapped Children and Young People. London, Routledge and Kegan Paul, 1978.
10. Anaise, J.: Periodontal disease and oral hygiene in a group of blind and sighted Israeli teenagers (14–17 years of age). J. Commun. Dent. Oral Epidemiol., *7*:353–356, 1971.
11. Ligh, R.Z.: The visually handicapped patient in dental practice. J. Dent. Handicapped, *4*(2):38–40, 1979.
12. Morsey, S.L.: Communicating with and treating the blind child. Dent. Hyg., *54*(6):288–290, 1980.
13. Yeadon, A.: Toward Independence: The Use of Instructional Objectives in Teaching Daily Living Skills to the Blind. New York, American Foundation for the Blind, 1974.
14. Willoughby, D.: A Resource Guide for Parents and Educators of Blind Children. Baltimore, National Federation of the Blind, 1979.
15. Clemens. C., and Taylor, S.: Toothbrushing to music. Dent. Hyg., *54*(3):125–126, 1980.
16. Lebowitz, E.: An introduction to dentistry for the blind. Dent. Clin. North Am., *18*(3):651–669, 1974.
17. Ball, R.O., Zucher, S.B., and Fretwell, L.D.: Teaching preventive dentistry to patients with impaired vision. J. Dent. Handicapped, *4*(1):23–25, 1978.

Chapter 4

ARTHRITIS AND RHEUMATIC DISEASES

"Arthritis" is a familiar term used to describe several disorders that cause pain in joints and connective tissue. Examination of mummies and human skeletal remains reveals that rheumatic diseases have affected mankind throughout history. Physicians of the eighteenth and nineteenth centuries began describing and differentiating the types of rheumatic diseases; the process of classifying the diseases was not completed, however, until this century.[1,2,3] Unfortunately, cures for these diseases do not exist; however, much can be done to improve the comfort of people with rheumatic diseases. A knowledge of arthritis will help the dental staff to make persons who experience this disease comfortable during oral care procedures.

DEFINITION AND INCIDENCE

More than one in every ten Americans, or about 21,000,000, have some form of arthritis. At any given time, about 3,500,000 Americans suffer from symptoms so debilitating that they are considered disabled.[4,5] Several forms of arthritis result in debilitation. Only the commonly observed forms of arthritis are presented in this chapter

The word arthritis is derived from the Greek words *arthron* (joint) and *itis* (inflammation), thus the description: inflamed joint. In our culture the word is used so widely that it covers all conditions (many without inflammation) that cause aching and pain in joints and connective tissues. The word *rheumatism* is often used in conjunction with arthritis. Rheumatism means a flowing out, or a secretion or discharge. The word originated centuries ago when physicians believed that joint disease was transmitted by the flow-

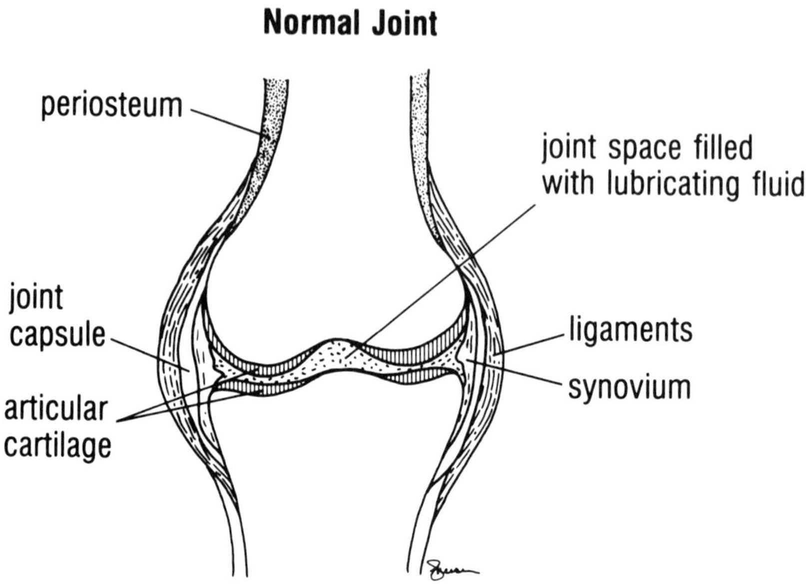

Fig. 4–1. A cross section of a normal joint.

ing of body fluids from one joint to another.[2] Today, the meaning of rheumatism is vague and covers a broad category of rheumatic disorders, including arthritis.[6] The word is used primarily to describe unexplained aches and pains in joints, muscles, and bones.

The common forms of arthritis are chronic in nature and tend to become worse if not treated. Once arthritis is diagnosed, treatment may continue throughout life. Swollen joints that are warm to the touch and painful to move indicate that inflammation is present. Inflammation is only an indication that tissue damage has occurred. Inflammation in a joint, however, generally results in further damage to the joint, and the damage caused by the inflammation leads to more inflammation. Continued damage to a joint results in stiffness and loss of the normal range of movement.[1,2]

ANATOMY OF A NORMAL JOINT

A review of the function and structure of a normal joint is helpful in understanding the nature of the disease. There are eight types of joints in the human body, each of which has a specific function. Those joints that are joined together loosely to allow movement (articulation) are joined by connective tissue.

Figure 4–1 represents the basic structure of all movable joints rather than a specific joint. As seen in the figure, the ends of the opposing bones (where the motion takes place) are covered with articular cartilage. The cartilage is strong yet flexible enough to absorb jolts sustained from bearing weight. Articular cartilage is a solid pad that does not have a blood supply or nerve tissue. Nutrients are obtained from fluids in the joint.

Typically, when a joint bears weight, the cartilage of one bone moves across the cartilage of the other bone. A thin membrane (the synovium) lines the surface of the interior of the joint. The function of this membrane is to secrete a small amount of fluid (synovial fluid) into the joint to provide lubrication. Tough fibrous tissue holds together and surrounds the joint, forming the joint capsule. Tendons attach to the joint capsule and allow the muscles to direct the movement of the joint. Without the interference of trauma or disease, joints can be expected to last a lifetime.[1,6]

CLASSIFICATION AND ETIOLOGY

Osteoarthritis

Osteoarthritis is the most commonly observed form of arthritis, affecting about 12,000,000 Americans.[5] Osteoarthritis is a degenerative process that occurs in joints that have a congenital defect or insufficient blood supply, or were at one time diseased or injured. Some sources identify osteoarthritis as the result of wear and tear that comes with age and the loss of tensile strength and fatigue resistance of cartilage.[7] The development of osteoarthritis was often blamed on increasing age. Age, however, is not the only factor responsible for wear and tear on joints. For example, some forms of employment (e.g., dock work, mining) place a great deal of stress on joints, which contributes to their wear.

Osteoarthritis is classified as (1) primary, with no specific cause, or (2) secondary, in which the cause is identified as trauma, infection, joint abnormality, or some other form of arthritis. Primary osteoarthritis is more generalized throughout the body and occurs more frequently in women. Secondary osteoarthritis usually occurs in the larger joints that bear weight, but can occur in any joint that is abused. The majority of diagnosed osteoarthritis cases are included in the first category.

The destructive process of osteoarthritis is the same no matter what the cause. The first step is the swelling and softening of the cartilage that covers the ends of the bones (Fig. 4–2). The swelling causes loss of density, creating cracking and pitting in the cartilage. The pitting can be minor or so serious that the cartilage sloughs off, causing the bones to contact and altering the shape of the joint. The loss of the cartilage causes strain at the margin of the bone. The bone ends become thick and calcium deposits appear,

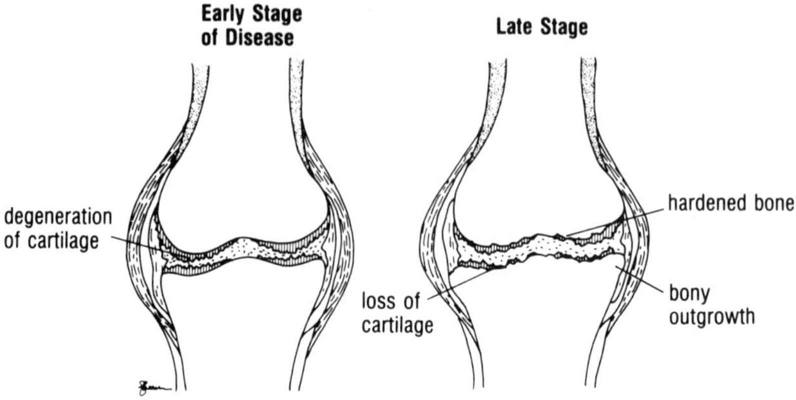

Fig. 4–2. The destructive process of osteoarthritis.

forming bony spurs (osteophytes). As the spurs gradually build up, they can break loose and interfere with joint movement. In advanced stages of osteoarthritis, the continued degeneration of cartilage and growth of spurs limit the normal action of the joint.

Osteoarthritis develops over a long period of time with periods of no progression. Symptoms may not appear until the disease process is advanced. The first symptom to appear is pain in the form of a mild aching and soreness, especially upon joint movement. Stiffness in the morning or after sitting for long periods is another common symptom. Cold, fatigue, and dampness can contribute to stiffness and pain. Typically, osteoarthritis does not severely limit the range of motion of affected joints, but the pain can contribute to decreased use of the affected joints, resulting in degeneration of supportive muscle and ultimately to poor posture.[2,3,8]

Rheumatoid Arthritis

Rheumatoid arthritis is the second most commonly observed form in the United States and the most serious, affecting about 5,000,000 adults and 250,000 children. The majority of patients in whom rheumatoid arthritis is diagnosed (about 70%) are between 25 and 54 years of age. Rheumatoid arthritis occurs at a female/male ratio of 3 to 1. The reason for the higher incidence in women is yet undetermined.[7] Rheumatoid arthritis usually causes severe disability by affecting several joints at the same time. The disease process typically progresses slowly, sometimes with periods of remission. Approximately 20% of adults with rheumatoid arthritis benefit from permanent remission of the disease; the remainder suffer with the disease throughout life.

Rheumatoid arthritis usually occurs in the small joints of the hands and feet. The disease process, however, can begin in wrist, ankle, elbow, or knee joints. In severe cases, the joints of the neck can be involved. Rheumatoid arthritis starts as an inflammation in the blood vessels supplying the synovium. As a result of the swelling, the synovium begins to enlarge and secretes more fluid, causing enlargement of the entire joint. This growth continues until the synovium overlaps the cartilage on the articulating surface of the bone. The synovium may grow between the two surfaces of cartilage, eventually causing cartilage degeneration. Additional loss occurs when enlarged blood vessels destroy cartilage from the bone side. If sufficient cartilage is lost, the bones will join, resulting in a stiff (ankylosed) joint (Fig. 4–3). Ankylosis is the most severe outcome of rheumatoid arthritis. The disease can be slowed or halted through treatment or remission.

Rheumatoid arthritis is difficult to distinguish from other diseases in the early stages. Diagnosis is accomplished through observation of the progress of the disease, x-rays, sedimentation rate of blood corpuscles, and tests for rheumatoid antibody. X-rays reveal joint destruction and track the progression of the disease.

The cause of rheumatoid arthritis is unknown. Currently two hypotheses are popular and are being researched.[1,7,8] Some researchers believe that rheumatoid arthritis is due to infection. Infected teeth and tonsils were once implicated as causative factors, resulting in many unnecessary extractions and tonsillectomies.[9] Others believe it is a result of autoimmunity, a process in which the body's autoimmune system malfunctions and the antibodies attack the body. Theoretically, during this process, proteins that are isolated in an enclosed space of the body break loose through injury

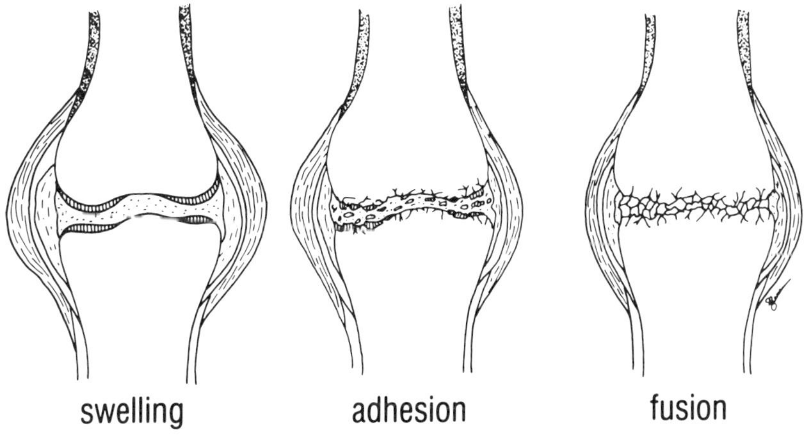

Fig. 4–3. The destructive process of rheumatoid arthritis.

and begin circulating. These proteins are unfamiliar to the body tissues, thereby promoting the formation of antibodies. The autoimmune hypothesis developed when many people with rheumatoid arthritis were noted to have a particular antibody in their blood. The antibody has been labeled the rheumatoid factor. The tests for the rheumatoid antibody are highly technical and usually are not performed unless other diagnostic procedures are inconclusive. Latest findings reveal that genetic markers have been identified that indicate a predisposition in certain people to develop this faulty immune reaction.[10]

Emotional or physical stress can aggravate or prolong recovery from the disease. Many patients report the onset or worsening of arthritis symptoms after the death of a loved one, divorce, or loss of employment. Investigators have examined possible connections between stress, diet, climate, and rheumatoid arthritis with no conclusive findings. A higher incidence rate of rheumatoid arthritis within families, however, has been noted.

One difference between the adult and childhood forms of this disease is that remission occurs in about 60 to 70% of children 10 years after onset. With adequate medical care, only 10% of affected children will be left with limitations of range and of motion. The remission rate for adults is only about 20%. The abnormal antibody found in most adults usually is not found in children.

Classification of childhood rheumatoid arthritis includes the polyarticular form and the systemic form. The polyarticular form can be identified by the number of joints affected (usually five or more), fever, rash, and anemia. The symptoms of the systemic form are similar to those of the polyarticular form, but are only part of a pattern of illness that includes high spiking fever (105° F) once or twice a day, enlarged lymph nodes, and an enlarged spleen. Permanent joint damage can be lessened by early diagnosis and treatment; the longer inflammation goes untreated, the greater the likelihood of permanent damage to the joints.[11]

Ankylosing Spondylitis

Ankylosing spondylitis is an inflammatory spinal arthritis that affects about 200,000 Americans. The process of degeneration is similar to that of rheumatoid arthritis. The disease process usually starts in the lower spine and is characterized by back stiffness in the morning. With disease progression, range of movement can be limited severely. Onset usually occurs between the ages 20 and 30. Recent research indicates that an almost equal number of males and females are affected, but symptoms in males are more severe.[1,2]

TREATMENT

Treatment for osteoarthritis includes: (1) monitoring the progression without intervening (no treatment); (2) nonoperative treatment (medications and/or support braces); (3) operative procedures (fusion of a joint, removal of foreign matter and nonfunctional structures of the joint, and implantation of artificial joints).

Aspirin is the most commonly prescribed medication for the treatment of osteoarthritis. Aspirin is considered the most reliable and least toxic of all antiarthritic drugs. It is the drug most likely to control symptoms and has the lowest risk for producing undesirable side effects. Splints and braces are used to provide support, reduce pressure from affected joints, and reduce the need for surgery.[6,8,12]

Treatment of rheumatoid arthritis can include the application of heat, hydrotherapy, bed rest, exercise, splinting, medications, and surgery. The treatment prescribed depends on the severity of symptoms and the progression of the degeneration. During the active state of the disease, many patients find that heat and hydrotherapy reduce pain and swelling. At times during the active state of the disease process, bed rest may be recommended to reduce movement and pressure on joints. Bed rest is sometimes supervised in a hospital to prevent the patient from assuming "comfortable" but deforming positions. Active exercise may be suggested during remission. The exercise is designed to maintain muscle tone and to avoid flexion deformities that result from lack of use. Splints are typically used as a form of treatment to protect joints rather than to limit motion.

Medications for people with rheumatoid arthritis include analgesics, anti-inflammatory drugs, and hypnotics. Typically, individuals with rheumatoid arthritis begin with aspirin. If they cannot tolerate aspirin or if it does not control the inflammation, other anti-inflammatory and immunosuppressive agents are used. Some of the more commonly prescribed drugs include gold compounds, phenylbutazone, adrenocortical steroids, and indomethacin. The drugs used in the treatment of rheumatoid arthritis depend on the individual's tolerance and the physician's preferences, and they are monitored closely for side effects.[8,12,13] Surgery is considered as a last resort. As in osteoarthritis, surgery of rheumatic joints includes the removal of foreign matter and inflamed synovial membrane and the implantation of artificial joints.[4,8]

Treatment for ankylosing spondylitis focuses on exercise to prevent postural deformities. The exercise program is quite rigorous and effective if followed. Medication may be prescribed to reduce stiffness, pain, and inflammation.

PSYCHOSOCIAL IMPLICATIONS

Persons who experience gradual limitation of movement and body deformities may become depressed, withdrawn, or frustrated if they are not well adjusted to their disability. Dealing with continual pain is also extremely stressful and fatiguing. These patients may want to avoid any tasks or procedures that produce or provoke even minimal pain. A sense of well being has a definite effect on the health of arthritic patients, so it is extremely important to reduce stress, allow independence with use of new skills, and maintain awareness of the patient's emotional as well as physical needs.

DENTAL MANAGEMENT

The major aspects of dental management include temporomandibular joint (TMJ) involvement, patient comfort, and the use of medications.

Osteoarthritis Implications

The most frequently observed symptoms are bruxism and occlusal imbalance. Clenching, luxation, subluxation, abnormal mandibular function and pain have also been reported in patients with osteoarthritis. The pathologic changes that occur in osteoarthritis can be identified as softening, erosion, and degeneration of the hyaline cartilage of the articular surface. Osteoarthritis of the TMJ rarely progresses to the point of osteophyte (bone spur) formation with resulting decreased joint space.[14,15]

Patient comfort involves relief of TMJ pain in the acute stage through the use of moist heat applied to the joint and the administration of anti-inflammatory medications. The patient with TMJ involvement may require the use of a mouth prop or frequent rests to lessen the strain of maintaining an open mouth. Patient comfort also includes modifications in the treatment plan to allow support of other body joints that may be severely involved. Joints not in use are less painful; therefore, sitting in the dental chair for a period of time should pose no problem. When hip, knee, or ankle joints are severely involved, some movement or exercise will be required before the patient attempts to stand. Arthritic patients should not be exposed to drafty or overly air-conditioned waiting rooms since the drafts cause stiffness and soreness. If medication is prescribed, the patient's physician should be consulted prior to administering the medication.[14,15]

Rheumatoid Arthritis Implications

Rheumatoid arthritis has been reported to affect the TMJ in 10 to 70% of observed patients. The wide range is due in part to the lack of standardization of diagnostic techniques and the stage of the arthritis being observed. The diagnosis of TMJ involvement in the beginning stages of rheumatoid arthritis is difficult.[16] Early symptoms of TMJ involvement include redness, tissue warmth, swelling, difficulty in movement, and pain upon chewing and opening. The process of TMJ joint destruction is the same as for other joints. As the disease progresses, the pain diminishes, a result of loss of mobility. Radiographic studies of TMJ with rheumatic arthritis reveal flattening of the anterior aspect of the condylar head, destruction of the articular surfaces, and clouding of the joint space, which indicates development of fibrotic tissue.[17]

Dental procedures should be modified to accommodate the symptoms of the patient. For example, in the initial stage of rheumatoid arthritis when joints are red, swollen, and tender to the touch, gentleness in approaching routine procedures is required. In the intermediate stage, movement of the affected joints is limited and difficult to accomplish because of associated pain. Support for affected joints with pillows or the use of soft restraints may be needed. Frequent rest periods with changes of position are necessary but can lengthen an appointment, an important consideration for appointment scheduling. Few patients with advanced rheumatoid arthritis can tolerate appointments longer than 20 to 30 minutes, even with support and changing of position. In order to take full advantage of tolerance levels, patients with intermediate and advanced stages of rheumatoid arthritis should not spend excessive time in the waiting room or in the dental chair.

As with osteoarthritis, patients may benefit from the application of moist heat to the TMJ or other joints that cause discomfort prior to their dental appointment. The use of mouth props can reduce patient fatigue and discomfort for persons with limited range of motion in the TMJ (Fig. 4–4). Limited oral access may necessitate compromises in diagnostic or treatment procedures (Fig. 4–5). In some cases, panoramic radiographs may be the only practical means of obtaining an x-ray. Adjustments in the instrumentation during periodontal debridements and restorative procedures may be necessary. Consequently, precise periodontal debridements may be impossible.

Most patients with intermediate to advanced stages of rheumatoid arthritis will be taking medication such as aspirin or sodium salicylates for pain and swelling. Steroids may also be given. One

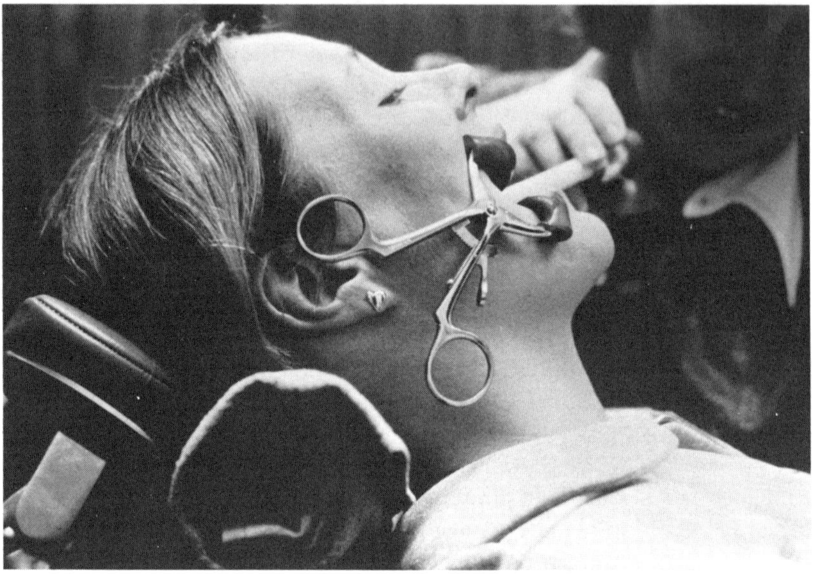

Fig. 4–4. The use of neck support and mouth prop can lengthen treatment time.

side effect of large doses of salicylates is a lowering of prothrombin levels in the blood. Deep scaling or extractions, therefore, may result in excessive bleeding. The attending physician should be consulted about the patient's bleeding time. Deep scaling procedures may have to be delayed. Anemia that is not ameliorated by medication or nutritional therapy may exist. Delayed healing after periodontal debridement or extraction is common in anemia.

Prolonged steroid therapy produces several side effects, including the body's dependency on the medication and the masking of inflammatory signs. To avoid serious problems with these patients, the physician should be consulted for possible adjustment of steroid therapy before and after dental treatment.

Antibiotics should be considered for any patient undergoing surgery during an acute arthritic phase. The swelling produced by an acute attack decreases the body's ability to combat infections.[9] Surgery for patients with severe TMJ involvement should be considered only as a last resort, and only when the patient's overall health is in jeopardy (e.g., inability to eat or TMJ ankylosis). Such surgery usually involves replacement of the TMJ.[18]

Since juvenile rheumatoid arthritis affects children in the developmental years, it interferes with dental growth and development. Inflammation of the TMJ in childhood and adolescence can slow or temporarily stop the growth of the mandible. This loss of condylar growth is not regained in later years. The physical appearance of these children can be altered, resulting in micrognathia or a beak-like appearance. Anterior open bite and crowding of mandibular anterior teeth have also been noted. Orthodontic treatment can lessen the effects of malocclusion resulting from the arthritis. Class II malocclusion is seen frequently, but not all children with TMJ involvement demonstrate malocclusion.[17]

Ankylosis Implications

Patients with ankylosing spondylitis typically present minimal management problems. Rarely are the TMJ or the vertebrae of the neck involved. If back support is provided and patients are allowed to change position frequently, they can withstand a normal appointment period.

PREVENTIVE MEASURES

Preventive procedures for patients with arthritis should focus on eliminating oral infection and adapting home care techniques to compensate for limited joint movement. Home care procedures may be compromised by limited oral opening and difficulty in reaching the mouth because of joint involvement of the hands, wrists, elbows, or shoulders. Insertion of a mouth prop during brushing may prevent patient fatigue and pain from maintaining an open jaw. If finger joints are involved, enlarging the handles of the toothbrush or floss holder or using an electric toothbrush may be

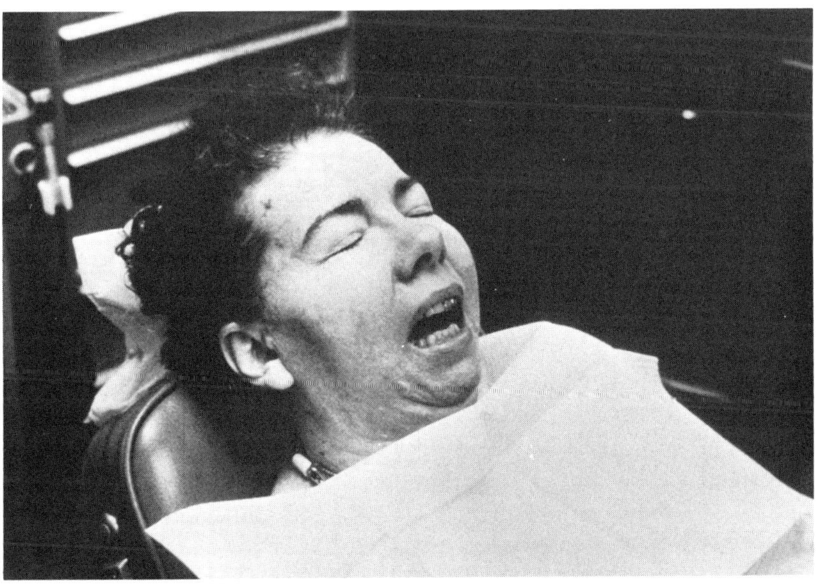

Fig. 4–5. Limited oral access due to rheumatoid arthritis of the temporomandibular joint.

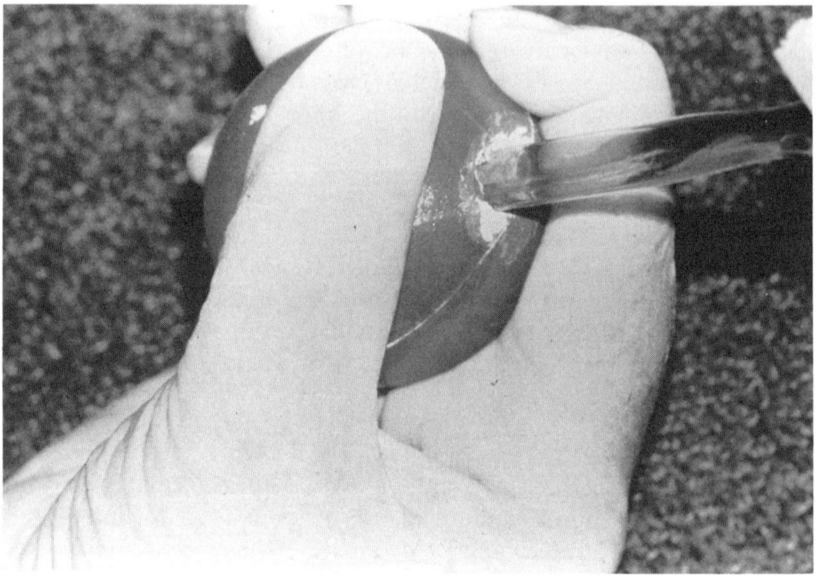

Fig. 4–6. Oral health aids will have to be modified when finger joints become severely involved.

helpful (Fig. 4–6). If elbow or shoulder joints are involved, extended or bent handles might be needed. The use of denture brushes mounted on suction cups will facilitate cleaning of dentures or removable partial dentures. Children with juvenile rheumatoid arthritis must be taught oral hygiene techniques early, particularly if the teeth are crowded or malocclusion leads to mouth breathing.

When oral hygiene is compromised, frequently rinsing the mouth with water helps to dislodge food particles. Fluoride rinses are also beneficial for reducing plaque pathogenicity. These procedures are particularly important if the patient is confined to bed and must rely on others for care. Consultation with the patient's physician or those who provide daily care can help ensure continuity of care. Patients receiving long-term medications should be made aware of the side effects of delayed healing and possible bleeding difficulties.

PATIENT SCENARIOS

Patient 1

Description

Mrs. J. is a 67-year-old woman who has been coming to your office for many years. She has osteoarthritis. She wears an upper denture and has many mobile mandibular teeth.

Anticipated Needs

—thorough soft tissue examination
—oral hygiene instruction
—periodontal debridement and root planing

Awareness Strategies

1. Would it be better to schedule her in the early morning or early afternoon?
2. What symptoms of arthritis might she present during the dental appointment?
3. What adaptations might be needed in instrumentation or positioning?
4. What difficulties might she have with home care?

Patient 2

Description

Mary F. is 35 years old and has rheumatoid arthritis in the intermediate stage. She can no longer work as a typist because of her condition and is presently seeking other employment. She has not been seen by a dentist for five years.

Anticipated Needs

—a thorough examination and x-rays
—periodontal debridement and oral hygiene instruction
—moderate amount of restorative treatment

Awareness Strategies

1. What might Mary's emotional status be? How might you approach her to make the dental visits more pleasurable?
2. What arthritis symptoms might she have?
3. Why might you want to restrict the number of x-rays taken in the dental office?
4. What factors might interfere with optimal home oral hygiene care?

Patient 3

Description

Jamie is a 14-year-old boy with childhood rheumatoid arthritis. He has never seen a dentist and is ashamed of his condition. He attends special classes for health-impaired adolescents.

Anticipated Needs

—complete examination and x-rays
—restorative treatment

—oral hygiene instruction and preventive procedures
—orthodontic consultation

Awareness Strategies

1. What oral manifestations do you expect of Jamie?
2. What information do you need to consider when scheduling Jamie for an appointment?
3. How will you make Jamie feel at ease in the dental setting?
4. How should you approach oral hygiene instruction with Jamie?

REFERENCES

1. Scott, J.: Arthritis and Rheumatism. New York, Oxford University Press, 1980.
2. Crain, D.: The Arthritis Handbook: A Patient's Manual of Arthritis, Rheumatism and Gout. New York, Exposition Press, 1971.
3. Sokoloff, L.: The Biology of Degenerative Joint Disease. Chicago, University of Chicago Press, 1969.
4. Swezey, R.: Arthritis: Rational Therapy and Rehabilitation. Philadelphia, W.B. Saunders, 1978.
5. Arthritis: The Basic Facts. New York, The Arthritis Foundation, 1976.
6. Adams, J.: Arthritis and Back Pain. Baltimore, University Park Press, 1972.
7. Rosenbaum, E.: Rheumatology: New Directions in Therapy. Garden City, N.Y., Medical Examination Publishers, 1979.
8. Roth, S.: New Directions in Arthritis Therapy. Littleton, Mass., PSG Publishing, 1980.
9. Sorenson, H.: Physically Handicapped. *In* Dentistry for the Handicapped Patient. Edited by A. Nowak. St. Louis, C.V. Mosby, 1976.
10. Harson, I.: Outwitting Arthritis. Berkeley, Creative Arts Book Co., 1980.
11. Miller, J.: Juvenile Rheumatoid Arthritis. *In* Physically Handicapped Children: A Medical Atlas for Teachers. Edited by E. Bleck and D. Nagel. New York, Grune & Stratton, 1975.
12. National Institute of Arthritis, Metabolism and Digestive Diseases: How to Cope with Arthritis. Bethesda, Maryland, NIH 76-1092, 1976.
13. Kay, A.: Adverse reactions to anti-rheumatic drugs: methods of monitoring. *In* Laboratory Tests in Rheumatic Disease: Standardization in Clinical Laboratory Investigation. Edited by D.C. Dumonde and M.W. Steward. Baltimore, University Park Press, 1979.
14. Guttenberg, S.: Arthritis disorders of the temporomandibular joint. Journal of the D.C. Dental Society, pp. 9–13, Winter, 1978.
15. Kreutziger, K., and Mahan, P.: Temporomandibular degenerative joint disease. Oral Surg. Oral Med., Oral Pathol., *49*(2):165–181, 1975.
16. Ogus, H.: Rheumatoid arthritis of the temporomandibular joint. Brit. J. Oral Surg., *12*:275–284, 1975.
17. Trenwith, J., and Beale, C.: Rheumatoid arthritis in the temporomandibular joint. NZ Dent. J., *973A*:195–199, 1977.
18. Morgan, D.: Surgical correction of temporomandibular joint arthritis. J. Oral Surg., *33*(10):766–773, 1975.

Chapter 5
LUNG DISORDERS

In the past, lung disorders implied infections such as tuberculosis and pneumonia, which were often fatal until the advent of antibiotics. Lung disorders today tend to be more chronic in nature. Typically, these include cystic fibrosis, asthma, bronchitis, and emphysema. As a group, these chronic pulmonary diseases are becoming more prevalent in the United States.

CYSTIC FIBROSIS

Cystic fibrosis is the most frequent cause of chronic lung disease in Caucasian children in the U.S. It affects children early in life, restricts normal development, and leads to an early death. Prior to the introduction of antibiotics, children born with cystic fibrosis usually died within the first two years of life. Recent advancements in treatment enable many of these children to live into their twenties and thirties. However, the regimen of treatment severely limits their physical activities.

Cystic fibrosis was first described in 1936 and recognized as a unique disease process affecting children in 1938. Originally observed in the pancreas, it was described as cystic fibrosis of the pancreas.[1,2,3] As new discoveries about the disease process have emerged, the name has been shortened. The disease affects many of the body's organ systems. The problems created by organ dysfunction and the treatments employed to lessen the effects of the disease have implications that affect delivery of dental care.

Incidence

Cystic fibrosis is an inherited disorder. Estimates of the incidence rate in the United States range from 1:1000 to 1:2000 live births. Two to five percent of the general population are carriers. Males and females are equally affected. Approximately 25% of

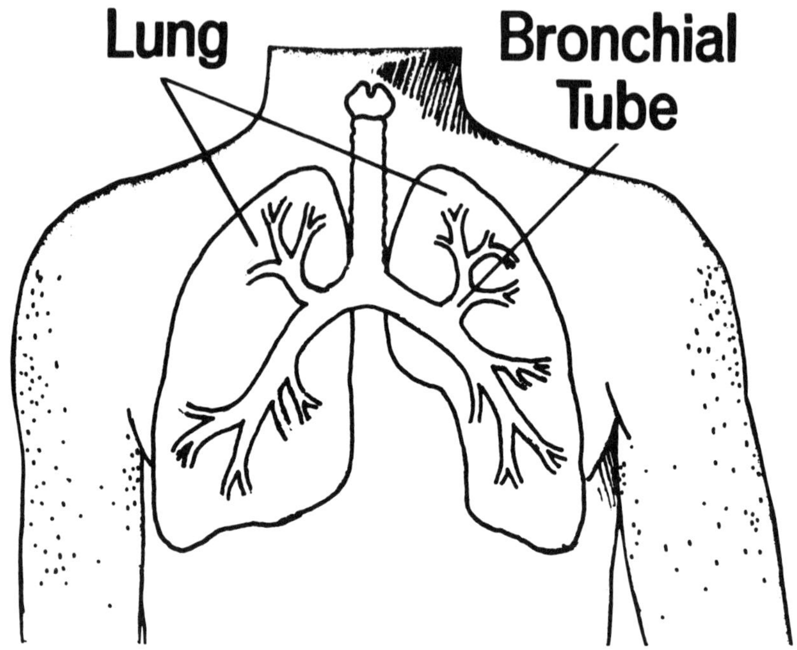

Fig. 5–1. Normal lungs.

siblings are affected, suggesting a recessive inheritance pattern.[3,4] Cystic fibrosis occurs most frequently in Caucasians of European lineage, and rarely in Orientals, Blacks, and Indians.[1,5]

Symptoms

Cystic fibrosis affects the exocrine glands, which secrete mucus, saliva, and sweat; the secretions produced are chemically or physically abnormal. In normal lungs (Fig. 5–1), mucus is secreted by cells in the lining of the bronchial tubes. The mucus catches dust and other inhaled foreign particles and removes them from the lungs by cilia which move the particles up to the trachea, where it is swallowed or expectorated. In cystic fibrosis, the mucus cannot move easily due to its abnormally thick, sticky consistency, so that it is retained in the bronchi. The mucous accumulations eventually interfere with oxygen exchange by partially obstructing or occluding individual bronchi. Partial obstruction allows the inhalation of air, but interferes with its exhalation. This phenomenon causes the barrel-chested appearance characteristic of many people who have cystic fibrosis and pulmonary diseases (Fig. 5–2).

Air trapped in the hyperinflated air sacs is absorbed into the blood, causing collapse of the sacs. Infection of small bronchial tubes is caused by the inability of the lungs to remove the inhaled material and excessive mucus, and by damaged air sacs. As a result, suppurative bronchitis, pneumonia, and obstructive emphysema are common among cystic fibrosis patients. Clubbing of the fingers and toes is also common in advanced cases. A decreased exercise tolerance and chronic, productive cough are characteristic. Even with treatment, recurrent hyperinflation and infection can lead to eventual death through ineffective carbon dioxide and oxygen exchange or anoxia.[3,4,6]

When cystic fibrosis is present, the pancreas is smaller, thinner, and firmer than usual. In the normal pancreas, the secretions of

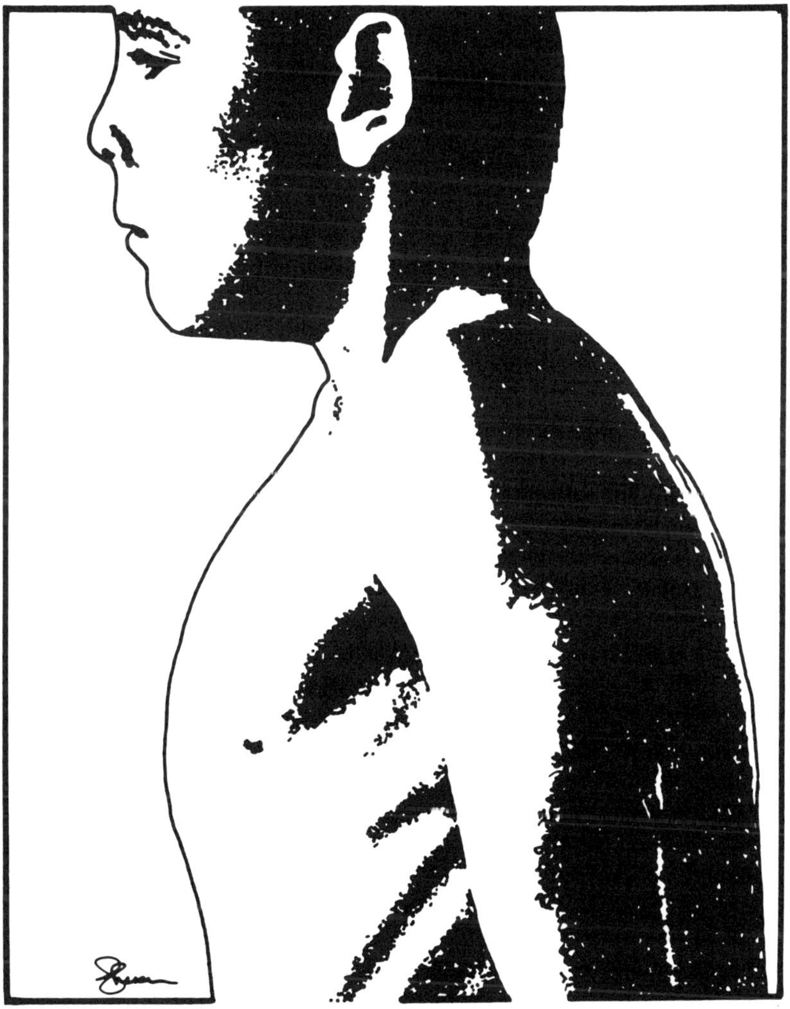

Fig. 5–2. Barrel-chested appearance common in people suffering from pulmonary diseases.

many small glands flow through small channels within the gland. The channels, like the tributaries of a river, join to form progressively larger ducts that terminate in the small intestine. In the intestines, pancreatic secretions assist in the metabolism of ketone bodies. The thickness of the secretions in individuals with cystic fibrosis blocks the pancreatic channels leading to the small intestine, causing eventual swelling and hardening (cystic formation) of the plugged gland and leading to its impaired metabolism and progressive deterioration.[4,7,8]

Nonmucus-producing glands (sweat or parotid glands) show no pathologic or histologic changes, but the chemical composition of their secretions is abnormal. Other findings include a small gallbladder in 20% of patients and localized areas of biliary obstruction in the liver, which sometimes lead to cirrhosis of the liver. Later complications often include diabetes mellitus, nasal polyps, rectal prolapse, heat prostration, and in males, sterility.

Diagnosis

Cystic fibrosis is initially suspected because of the symptoms manifested. These include delays in physical development, chronic respiratory illness, or foul smelling stools. The delays in physical development occur partly from inadequate metabolism caused by decreased levels of the pancreatic enzymes trypsin and chymotrypsin. Tryptinic activity for proper digestion is absent in over 80% of patients. Fecal examination usually reveals an increase in free fatty acids. Chest x-rays, as well as tracking the number, length, and severity of pulmonary infections, can assist in establishing a preliminary diagnosis.[9]

Cystic fibrosis is not easy to diagnose. The respiratory symptoms parallel those of bronchitis and asthma, while intestinal irregularities can resemble other intestinal disorders. The discovery of high levels of sodium in the perspiration of children with cystic fibrosis led to the development of the "sweat test" for determining electrolyte levels. This test helps to identify individuals who have cystic fibrosis, but cannot distinguish carriers of the disease.[4] A definitive diagnosis should be based on the following criteria: increased electrolyte concentration of perspiration, absence of pancreatic enzymes, chronic pulmonary involvement, and family history of the disorder.

Treatment

The exact cause of cystic fibrosis is not known, nor is there a cure. Treatment is primarily interceptive in nature and focuses on:

1. control of pulmonary infection

2. maintenance of nutrition for optimal growth and development
3. prevention or restoration of abnormal salt loss

Antibiotics, such as penicillin, streptomycin, clindamycin, dicloxacillin, or tetracycline are used to intercept and eliminate lung infections. Emphasis is placed on maintaining the lungs as mucus-free as possible. Aerosol inhalants are used to expand the bronchial tubes to maintain an open airway, and to increase hydration of the mucus to facilitate expectoration. Mist tents may be used at night to help thin the mucus. Mucus drainage is also facilitated by the technique of postural drainage: the person is positioned to promote drainage of the lungs while the chest is vibrated and massaged to dislodge the secretions.

Treatment is designed to alleviate digestive problems through dietary control and dietary supplements. Diets usually contain reduced total fat with increased calories and proteins. Powdered enzyme supplements (extract of animal pancreas) and vitamin and mineral supplements are included to offset the body's inability to process these nutrients. Regulation of salt intake is important in warm weather and during excessive exercise to avoid heat exhaustion due to salt loss.[1,4] In spite of these dietary modifications, linear growth and bone maturation are depressed, resulting in a thin body stature. The gaunt, young-looking body appearance, in addition to delayed puberty, can create self-image problems for adolescents, necessitating some form of professional counseling. An individually tailored program of physical activities can maintain and improve stamina.

The concept of disease prevention also includes genetic counseling for the family. Since carriers of cystic fibrosis cannot be identified, genetic counseling focuses on explaining to parents the probabilities of producing another child with cystic fibrosis and the probabilities of the siblings being carriers.[10] The development of a test to identify carriers continues to be a major goal of research.

Psychosocial Implications

The prospect of an early death, the cost of medical and supportive treatment, the reality of parenting a frail child, and the trauma of recurrent illnesses, along with the sympathy and guilt felt by most parents for these children, tend to produce an abnormal and stressful home environment. If the child and the illness dominate the home environment, all family members can be affected adversely. Health care professionals may encounter a variety of responses from family and patient, including denial, anxiety, guilt, resentment, hostility, indifference, or depression. Many families, on the other hand, demonstrate a positive outlook and lead relatively normal lives. Late adolescence may be a particularly difficult time for family and patients as they cope with decisions regarding social interactions, school, choice of a career, and advancing complications.

Families of a child with cystic fibrosis generally are served by a team of specialists, including physicians, nurses, nutritionists, and social workers. Consultation with these team members often facilitates treatment planning by providing insight into the family's behavior and knowing which member of the family the patient responds to best. Words or behavior that triggers negative or fearful responses can be identified to avoid introducing unintentional stress for the patient.

Dental Implications

Most patients with cystic fibrosis have had a lot of exposure to medical environments. Their reaction to the dental environment may be influenced greatly by these other experiences. Apprehension about specific medical procedures may be directly transferred to dental procedures. Oral procedures evoke fears of interfering with optimal airway function and may be threatening.

Cystic fibrosis patients have a lower caries rate, less plaque accumulation, less gingivitis, and increased calculus deposits. These findings are probably due to alterations in saliva composition, decreased saliva flow, prolonged antibiotic therapy, and the possible effects of the pancreatic enzyme replacement that is added to the diet.[9,11,12,13] The increased deposition of calculus has been attributed to the higher concentration of protein, calcium and phosphorus in the saliva.[14]

Cystic fibrosis often results in enlargement of the submaxillary and sublingual glands, which secrete a more viscous saliva at a lower rate than normal.[8,14] This altered flow rate and consistency can greatly impair the patient's ability to wear oral appliances comfortably. The "dry mouth" sensation can be unpleasant and also contribute to dryness and cracking of the lips.

Discoloration of the teeth in both primary and permanent dentition is common, although it does not affect the structure of the teeth. The staining is generally due to ongoing or prolonged antibiotic therapy or impaired oxygenation due to chronic lung obstruction (Fig. 5–3). Tetracycline is incorporated into the dentin during tooth development, and the severity of the discoloration does not appear to be related to dosage or the length of time the medication is taken.[15]

Mouth breathing as a result of an occluded nasal cavity or maxillary sinus from recurrent infections produces a high incidence of open bite malocclusion.

Dental Management

Because of their susceptibility to upper respiratory infections, children with cystic fibrosis should not be scheduled for appointments during the winter months when other children with colds might be sitting in the waiting room. Appointments may also have to be scheduled in the late afternoon or during school vacations to allow the patient to attend as much classroom time as possible between bouts of illness. Consultation with the physician should occur early, so that scheduling and treatment planning decisions can be based on a thorough analysis of the individual's needs and constraints. Patient comfort is most important during dental procedures that potentially impair airway exchange and interfere with expectoration, producing undue stress and a feeling of suffocation. A rubber dam should be used whenever possible, but it may have to be removed occasionally. During other procedures that do not require a rubber dam, the oral cavity should remain as uncluttered as possible. Frequent water rinses and evacuation are helpful, especially when using prophy paste, which tends to thicken saliva. Placing the chair in a more upright position may decrease the patient's anxiety and labored breathing, and facilitate coughing, which dislodges mucus. Respiratory depressants such as narcotics or tranquilizers should be avoided.

Treatment of staining to improve an esthetic appearance is accomplished through vital tooth bleaching, acid etch, laminate ve-

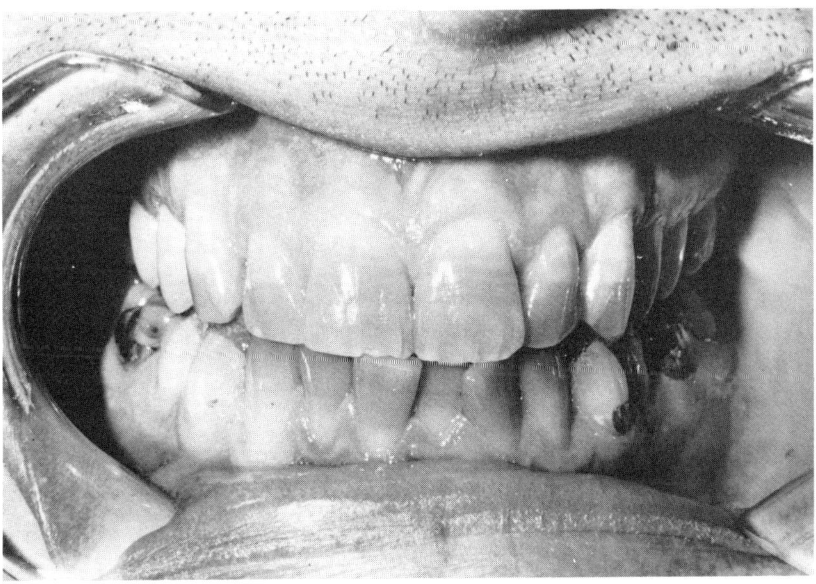

Fig. 5–3. Staining of teeth due to antibiotic therapy.

neer covering, or full coverage crowns.[16,17] The placement of full coverage crowns is often expensive and not feasible for families with limited finances.[18]

Preventive Measures

Although individuals with cystic fibrosis reportedly accumulate less plaque due to salivary changes and treatment regimens, oral hygiene maintenance is still important. Frequent brushing should be encouraged to ensure healthy gingiva and to decrease breath problems arising from accumulated bacteria and mucus on the tongue and tissues. The importance of toothbrushing and flossing can be introduced as (1) an important component of oral esthetics, (2) a procedure for decreasing oral odors, and (3) a mechanism for preventing oral infection, which could lead to other infections. These concepts are sometimes accepted more readily if reinforced by other members of the health care team, particularly the physician, nurse, and nutritionist. Dental information and written materials should be provided to these professionals and to the patients. Clinics that meet regularly and serve as a regional resource for patients with cystic fibrosis often have a dental hygienist to perform oral screenings, facilitate dental referrals, and provide dental health education to patients and their families.

Other preventive procedures, such as pit and fissure sealants and fluoride applications, are also important to the patient's health. Thorough, more frequent debridements may be necessitated by abnormal calculus accumulations. Patients may benefit from a short recall visit every two to three months for a plaque check and scaling procedures. Although dietary counseling is an integral part of preventive dentistry, dietary recommendations should be closely coordinated with the dietary regimen prescribed by the other health care providers.

Because of the nature of the illness, patients may consider dental health a low priority issue. Limited finances may negate frequent

TABLE 5–1. Common Precipitating/Aggravating Factors for Asthmatic Attacks

Antigens	Other Precipitating Factors
Dust	Weather
Mold	Exercise
Pollen	Emotional encounters
Animal dander	Infections
Household sprays	Menstrual cycle
Smoke	Stress
Air pollutants	

office visits or esthetic restoration of discolored teeth. Parental reactions to a frail, sick child may hamper referrals for dental care or interfere with optimal provision of home care. Frequent bouts of illness may postpone needed dental treatment. Children and adolescents who are depressed and exhibit low self-esteem may resist any attempts to promote self-maintenance skills such as toothbrushing. Low-key instruction and dental health education is sometimes more effective with these patients than idealistic, intensive preventive programs.

BRONCHIAL ASTHMA

Bronchial asthma is a generalized destructive disease of the airway characterized by pulmonary insufficiency due to pulmonary obstruction. Obstruction may be due to muscle constriction, edema, blood vessel dilation, or hypertrophy of the bronchial walls. Bronchial asthma affects 2.5% of the general population. Initial presentation of symptoms occurs most often in the first five years of life.[19] Bronchospasms are triggered by various factors, some of which cause an antigen-antibody response. The antigen-antibody reaction results when an antigen such as those listed in Table 5–1 enters the body, usually through the respiratory passages, and stimulates the production of an antibody. These antibodies circulate within serum, causing enzymatic reactions including the release of mediators, the most common of which is histamine. Histamine then produces increased bronchial secretions and edema of the mucous membranes and bronchial tract. People with asthma are considered more highly reactive than the general population to these mediators or to irritants. Stress factors such as emotional encounters or exercise can also precipitate the same reaction.

Symptoms

Symptoms occur in the lower and upper respiratory tracts and are observed in terms of their seasonal timing, frequency, and persistence. Common symptoms are wheezing, dyspnea, coughing, chest pain, sputum production, sneezing, runny nose, hoarseness, and fatigue. Syncope, respiratory failure, and cyanosis are more serious symptoms and can constitute a medical emergency called "status asthmaticus." Facial (sinus) pain, conjunctivitis, and otitis media are also common.[20,21,22]

Treatment

The medical management of asthma involves the treatment of the symptoms and the prevention of factors that trigger attacks. Symptoms are generally treated through the use of antihistamines (e.g., theophylline), decongestants, and bronchial dilators such as isoproterenol (Isuprel) and epinephrine (Primatene mist). Steroids are used as a last resort. The management of precipitating or aggravating factors usually requires the assistance of a health professional trained to identify problems or specific behavior patterns that trigger attacks. Management regimens include the avoidance of precipitating factors (no smoking), management or elimination of environmental factors (immaculate housecleaning, no pets, moving to a dry, pollen-free climate), dietary control (avoidance of allergenic foods), and relaxation techniques.

Psychosocial Implications

As with persons who have cystic fibrosis, the maintenance of adequate breathing is a major concern for persons with asthma. Fear of suffocation and stress from worrying about and dealing with the unpredictability of future attacks create stress within the family. Vacation plans may be dictated by geographic and seasonal limitations imposed by dust, pollutants, and pollen, or interrupted by a series of attacks. Living arrangements often involve the expenditure of extensive parental energy toward meticulous housecleaning to avoid the accumulation of dust and molds. The opportunity to own and be responsible for raising a pet may also be denied. Favorite foods may be restricted for the patient while other family members are allowed to eat them. Families who do not adhere strictly to the individualized therapy plan, particularly medication regimes, risk having to deal with severe attacks for which they are not prepared, thus jeopardizing the person's life and emotional status. Poor school attendance due to frequent illness and attacks can also lead to social and educational problems.

Dental Management

The following information should be obtained from dental patients who report a history of asthma: precipitating factors, current treatment regimen, degree of control or prevention achieved by treatment, and other allergies or medical problems.

Typically, individuals with chronic asthma do not present unusual problems in dental management or treatment and do not require adaptations to their home care program. Appointments may have to be scheduled during vacations or after school if a child has missed many school days. If the patient appears fearful in the dental environment, measures should be taken to alleviate the anxiety and lessen the strain of the appointment. Kinsman and associates suggest that anxiety can be best reduced by identifying the specific stressor. If the stressor is fear of the overall environment, a "tell-show-do" sequence can help to desensitize the patient.[23] Tell the patient the purpose or function of a procedure or equipment, demonstrate its function or purpose, and allow him or her to explore the instrument when practical. The desensitization process can begin with the operation of the dental chair. However, if the fear or anxiety is focused on injections or cavity preparations, replace the tell-show-do procedure with distractors. Discussing the patient's hobbies or interests while using a topical anesthetic, blocking the patient's view of the syringe by keeping it out of his or her line of vision, and depositing the anesthetic slowly often result in a less traumatic experience for the patient. Patients can also be encouraged to utilize their own relaxation regimens prior to and during the appointment to manage stress. Nitrous oxide should be used only after consulting with the physician. Oral agents such as chloral hydrate and hydroxyzine pamoate are the most practical agents of choice for sedation; narcotics should be avoided because they may cause a release of histamine.[15] Adverse drug interactions between erythromycin and theophylline have also been reported.[24]

Dental procedures that require general anesthesia may not be advisable for the reasons listed in Table 5–2.

If the asthmatic patient is properly prepared for an appointment and if the environment is free of antigens to which the patient is sensitive, it is unlikely that an emergency will develop. If the patient carries a nebulizer to the appointment, leave it in a conspicuous place near the dental chair in case it is needed. Stop all procedures and place the patient in an upright position if bronchospasms begin to occur. If the symptoms do not subside on their own or with the patient's usual medications, medical assistance may have to be summoned. The patient should be taken to an emergency room if symptoms do not subside in 20 minutes.[20]

BRONCHITIS

Symptoms

Bronchitis is frequently associated with allergies or chronic infections of the sinus or nasopharynx. Bronchitis may be an acute or

TABLE 5–2. Contraindications for General Anesthesia

1. Emotional stress of the procedure may precipitate an acute attack.
2. Patient's medications can interact adversely with the anesthetic agents.
3. Anesthetic agents may provoke an attack.
4. Airway stimulation may cause reflex bronchospasm.
5. Artificial ventilation may be inadequate for the patient who experiences severe bronchospasms.
6. Problems in removing secretions may result in postoperative pneumonia.
7. Inadequate respiratory reserve may hinder the patient's ability to recover from the operation and the anesthesia.[19]

chronic inflammation of the bronchial tree accompanied by a loss of elasticity of the lungs. Chronic bronchitis usually develops from prolonged lung infection or irritation by chemical and physical agents, such as coal dust and air pollution.[25] Hyperplasia and hyperactivity of the mucous glands results in persistent, sometimes paroxysmal, coughing with the production of a mucopurulent sputum.

Treatment

Medical management is similar to other respiratory disorders, usually involving postural drainage, treatment of allergic symptoms, and administration of antibiotics for bacterial infections. Unlike asthma, bronchodilators such as isoproterenol (Isuprel) do not alleviate symptoms.

Dental Management

Provide the patient with opportunities for coughing during dental procedures. If nitrous oxide analgesia is considered, the patient's physician should be consulted prior to treatment. The patient should be encouraged to brush more frequently or to use mouthrinse to avoid the accumulation of mucus and plaque.

EMPHYSEMA

Emphysema is the most frequently observed chronic disease of the lungs in adults. The exact etiology cannot be determined in each individual, but polluted air, cigarette smoking, and dust seem to be causative factors. Patients with chronic obstructive lung disease often develop both chronic bronchitis and emphysema.[26] Even in early stages of the disease, over 50% of the lung capacity may be destroyed before the effects are noticed.

Symptoms

Emphysema is characterized by abnormal dilation of the air spaces distal to the terminal bronchioles, resulting from the destruction of air sacs within the lungs. As the alveolar sacs lose their elasticity and tear, they leave behind air spaces that resist air flow; consequently breathing becomes progressively more difficult. With the loss of significant lung capacity, the lungs swell with trapped carbon dioxide. The patient may then exhibit a hyperinflated chest that is generally in an inspiratory or barrel-chested position. As more air sacs are destroyed, the heart works harder to pump the oxygen-deficient blood to the body tissues. Typical symptoms include wheezing, chronic coughing, dyspnea, and sometimes cyanosis of the lips and fingertips. If emphysema occurs in conjunction with chronic bronchitis, the cilia of the bronchial tree are damaged or destroyed, resulting in impaired removal of mucus; therefore, mucus must be coughed up and expectorated. The strain produced by this process may further destroy air sacs. Although a progressive disease, emphysema does respond to management such as avoidance of irritants, prevention of lung infections, oxygen therapy, and exercise.[7,27]

Dental Management

Patients with emphysema should not be scheduled during cold weather or remain in waiting rooms with other patients who are smoking or have upper respiratory infections. Afternoon appointments are preferable, since patients will have had time to carry out procedures that clear the tracheobronchial tree. Patients who experience severe breathing problems may prefer a more upright chair position and the avoidance of rubber dams or other materials that block their airway. As with the other respiratory disorders, barbiturates and narcotics should be avoided because they depress the respiratory center. Anesthetics such as nitrous oxide should be avoided, since high oxygen concentrations can lead to depressed respiration.

PATIENT SCENARIOS

Patient 1

Description

Johnny is six years old and has cystic fibrosis. His teeth are stained and his mother has scheduled an appointment for him. When they arrive at your office, Johnny is clinging to his mother and she seems anxious.

Anticipated Needs

—screening examination
—home care instructions
—bleaching or etching procedures

Awareness Strategies

1. How can you relieve the mother's stress and help Johnny relax?
2. What information does the mother need about the stained teeth?
3. What steps can you take to assist them both to meet home care needs?
4. What will you discuss about Johnny's diet?

Patient 2

Description

Frances is 13 years old and has had asthma since childhood. She has an appointment in your office for the first time.

Anticipated Needs

—screening
—radiographs
—home care instructions
—specific dental procedures

Awareness Strategies

1. What information do you need about Frances' condition?
2. How will you attempt to ensure that Frances will be comfortable in the dental environment?
3. What information do you need about Frances' medications?
4. What precautions will you take if Frances begins wheezing during treatment?

Patient 3

Description

Mr. Brown is a 63-year-old retired fireman. He has had emphysema for several years. He has been a regular patient, and this is an annual recall. Your office is in Kirby, Montana.

Anticipated Needs

—prophylaxis
—select radiographs
—select procedures
—home care instructions

Awareness Strategies

1. When would you schedule Mr. Brown for his appointment?
2. What precautions will you take to prevent coughing while you are taking radiographs?
3. How will you plan for Mr. Brown's arrival at the office?
4. How can you assure Mr. Brown's comfort during the dental procedures?

REFERENCES

1. Anderson, C.: Pancreatic disease in childhood. *In* The Exocrine Pancreas. Edited by J. Howat and H. Sarles. Philadelphia, W.B. Saunders, 1979.
2. Burton, I.: The Family Life of Sick Children. London, Routledge and Kegan Paul, 1975.
3. Harvey, B.: Cystic Fibrosis. *In* Physically Handicapped Children: A Medical Atlas for Teachers. Edited by E. Bleck and P. Nagel. New York, Grune & Stratton, 1975.
4. Anderson, C., and Goodchild, M.: Cystic Fibrosis Manual of Diagnosis and Management. Oxford, Blackwell Scientific Publications, 1976.
5. Schaap, T., and Cohen, M.: A proposed model for the inheritance of cystic fibrosis. *In* Cystic Fibrosis: Projections into the Future. Edited by J. Mangos and J. Talamo. New York, Stratton Intercontinental Medical Book Corp., 1976.
6. Mangos, J., and Talamo, R.: Fundamental Problems of Cystic Fibrosis and Related Diseases. New York, Intercontinental Medical Book Corp., 1973.
7. Adams, R., Daniel, A., McCubbin, J., and Rullman, L.: Games, Sports and Exercises for the Physically Handicapped. ed. 2. Philadelphia, Lea & Febiger, 1982.
8. Thompson, H.: Cystic fibrosis: a review. J. Nebraska Dent. Assoc., *50*:6–8, 1973.
9. Blacharsh, C.: Dental aspects of patients with cystic fibrosis: a preliminary clinical study. J. Am. Dent. Assoc., *95*(1):106–110, 1977.
10. Denning, R., Muriel, G., and Mohr, I.: Psychological and social aspects of cystic fibrosis. *In* Cystic Fibrosis: Projections into the Future. Edited by J. Mangos and J. Talamo. New York, Stratton Intercontinental Medical Book Corp., 1976.
11. Negon, E., and Liljemark, W.: Prevalence of certain plaque organisms in patients with cystic fibrosis: a clinical microbiological investigation. J. Dent. Res., *59*(11):1993–1994, 1980.
12. Primosch, R.: Tetracycline discoloration, enamel defects, and dental caries in patients with cystic fibrosis. J. Oral Surg., *50*(4):301–308, 1980.
13. Jagels, A., and Sweeney, E.: Oral health of patients with cystic fibrosis and their siblings. J. Dent. Res., *55*(6):991–996, 1976.
14. Epstein, N., et al.: Standardization of a new minor salivary gland collecting procedure for the diagnosis of cystic fibrosis. J. Dent. Children, *41*(6):461–464, 1974.
15. Sanger, R.G., and Bystrom, E.G.: Oral manifestations of immunologic and respiratory diseases. *In* Pediatric Dentistry: Scientific Foundations and Clinical Practice. Edited by R.E. Stuart. St. Louis, C.V. Mosby, 1982.
16. Posnick, W.R., and Fergal, R.J.: Cystic fibrosis and its dental implications. J. Dent. Handicapped, *5*(1):21–23, 1980.
17. Cohen, S., and Parkins, F.M.: Bleaching tetracycline-stained teeth. Oral Surgery, *29*:465–471, 1972.
18. Ettinger, R., and Pinkham, J.: Modifications in restorative dentistry for the handicapped patient. *In* Dentistry for the Handicapped Patient. Edited by A.J. Nowak. St. Louis, C.V. Mosby, 1976.
19. Gershwin, M.E. (ed.): Bronchial Asthma: Principles of Diagnosis and Treatment. New York, Grune & Stratton, 1981.
20. Dworin, A., and Gobetti, J.: Medical emergencies in dental practice. Part IV: The dyspneic patient. J. Michigan Dent. Assoc., *61*:347–350, 1979.
21. Strauss, S.: Management of the allergic patient. Florida Dent. J., *4*:15, 1974.
22. Crawford, L., Duncan, J., and Vanderpool, G.: The allergic child: special considerations in dentistry. *In* Dentistry and the Allergic Patient. Edited by C. Frazier. Springfield, Ill., Charles C Thomas, 1973.
23. Kinsman, R., Dirks, J., Jones, N., and Dahlen, N.: Anxiety reduction in

asthma: four catches to general application. Psychosom. Med., *43*:397–405, 1980.
24. Walker, J., and Hendeles, L.: The interaction of erythromycin and theophylline in the asthmatic dental patient. JADA, *99*:995–996, 1979.
25. Ogilvie, A., Stang, C., Leggat, P., and Newell, D.: A Ten Year Study of Chronic Bronchitis in the North East of England. Edinburgh, Churchill Livingstone, 1973.
26. Little, J.W., and Falace, D.A.: Pulmonary disease. *In* Dental Management of the Medically Compromised Patient. Edited by J.W. Little and D.A. Falace. St. Louis, C.V. Mosby, pp. 88–93, 1980.
27. Reid, L.: The Pathology of Emphysema. London, Lloyd Luke (Medical Book) Ltd., 1967.

Chapter 6

SPINAL CORD INJURIES

The loss of mobility and body function associated with traumatic injury to the spine entails a sudden and dramatic change in life style.[1] This suddenness, severity, and permanence of the change in life style has prompted the development of special rehabilitation programs for people with traumatic spinal cord injury. Rehabilitation programs strive to help these individuals adjust to their limitations, capitalize on their abilities, and establish realistic life goals. Yet society often becomes more intrigued with the adaptive devices, body supports, and wheelchairs than the individuals themselves. A personal, humanistic approach is important in normalizing the dental management of these patients.

INCIDENCE AND ETIOLOGY

The prevalence of spinal cord injury is reportedly between 150,000 and 200,000 people in the U.S. Approximately 70% of people with such injuries are below the age of 40; only about 15 to 20% are women. Fifty percent of the injuries result directly or indirectly from automobile or motorcycle accidents. Occupational accidents account for another 19 to 26%, while sporting accidents (primarily diving, trampoline, and football) account for another 18%. Other accidents, such as gunshot wounds or falls, account for the remainder.[2,3]

New cases of spinal cord injuries are estimated to range between 4,500 and 10,000 per year.[4,5] Many of these injuries could be avoided by proper adherence to safety measures, such as use of safety belts in automobiles.

REVIEW OF ANATOMY

The spinal cord and vertebral column comprise the spinal column (Fig. 6–1). The spinal cord is composed of nerve fibers and cells

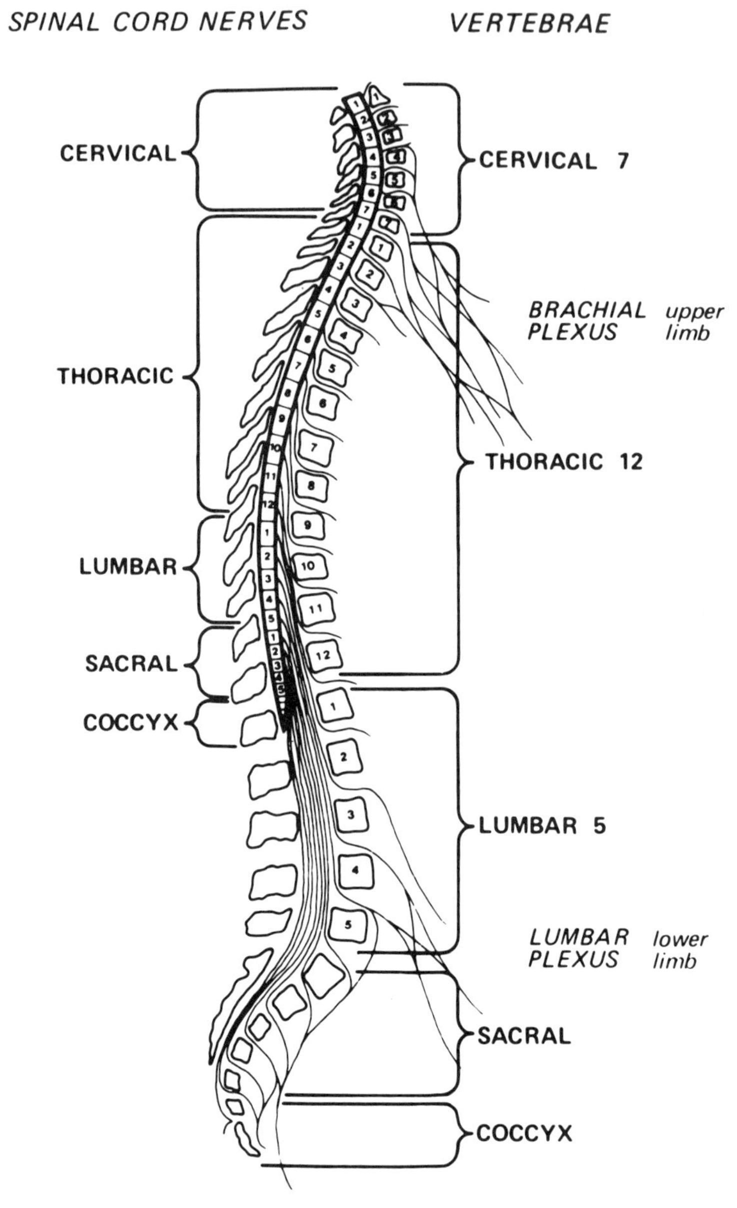

Fig. 6–1. Side view of the spinal column and the spinal cord indicating how the nerve roots emerge from the spinal cord to form the nerves to the limbs and organs. Note that the spinal cord ends at the level of the first or second lumbar vertebra. The confluence and rejoining of the nerve roots from the cervical area form the brachial plexus, which evolves into the major nerves of the upper limb; similarly, the nerves from the lower lumbar and sacral roots converge and reform to form the major nerves of the lower limb. (Reproduced by permission from Bleck, E.E. Anatomy: Basic Parts and Terms of the Nervous and Musculoskeletal Systems. *In* Physically Handicapped Children: A Medical Atlas for Teachers. Edited by E.E. Bleck, and D.A. Nagel. New York, Grune & Stratton, 1975.)

that descend from the brain and branch at 31 paired sites along the spinal column to reach all body parts. The consistency of the spinal cord is similar to that of a ripe banana. The function of the spinal cord is to provide a center for reflex actions and to act as a pathway for nerve impulses to and from the brain.[3,4,5,6]

The vertebral column contains irregularly shaped bones (vertebra) that are held together by ligaments and separated by discs. The vertebral column is capable of limited movement. The function of the vertebral column is to provide support for the body and to protect the spinal cord.

The spinal column contains four distinct curves. Two of the curves (thoracic and sacral) appear early in fetal development and are termed primary curves. The cervical curve appears late in fetal development; the lumbar curve appears as a child learns to walk. The vertebral column is divided into four sections, each corresponding to one of the curves.

DEFINITION AND CLASSIFICATION

Injury to the spinal cord occurs when all or a portion of the vertebral column undergoes fracture, dislocation, hyperextension, hyperflexion, rotation, or compression. Although injury can occur anywhere along the spinal column, it occurs most often in the cervical and lumbar curves.[3] Damage to the cord is usually due to disruption of any of the three arteries that supply the cord, which kills nerve cells supplied by the arteries. Some fractures and dislocations do not damage the cord; others put physical pressure on the cord, which also causes nerve cells to die. Paralysis occurs when the cord is severely traumatized, usually because of lack of blood supply to the nerve cells and pressure (swelling and bleeding) on the cord. Without access to the control center of the brain, body parts below the site of damage cannot function. Paralysis affects both motion and sensation. If the damage occurs in the thoracic, lumbar, or sacral portion of the vertebral column, paraplegia (paralysis of the legs and lower part of the trunk) results. If the damage is high in the cervical portion, quadriplegia/tetraplegia (paralysis of all four limbs and trunk) occurs.

The most commonly cited classification systems of spinal cord injury are those used in the United States and Europe. The first classification system describes the level of damage at the site on the vertebral column that is the last intact portion of the spinal cord. An example of a frequent injury would be C6 (cervical, sixth vertebra) (Fig. 6–1). The Asian-American Spinal Injury Association and the International Society of Paraplegia describe the most distant uninvolved cord segment along with the skeletal site of damage. This difference in classification seems minor, but cord damage can occur above or below the level of bone injury and may not be symmetrical. Consequently, two patients with a C6 injury can suffer different limitations.[3,5,6]

Not all spinal cord injuries result in complete spinal cord damage. For example, the cord can be partially damaged or compressed on the anterior aspect, leaving the posterior intact. In cases of incomplete lesions, some muscle recovery may occur in a few days or months after the injury. Neurologic recovery depends upon the severity and location of the injury to the cord and whether correct emergency procedures were followed at the scene of the accident. Many people suffer permanent spinal cord damage due to well intentioned but inappropriate first aid.[2,7,8] If any such damage is suspected, the injured person should not be moved or allowed to move until trained personnel arrive.

PSYCHOSOCIAL IMPLICATIONS

Patients with spinal cord injuries usually progress through various identifiable stages of grief after their accident. Shock, denial, reaction, mobilization, and coping are fluid stages of the grieving process, with patients experiencing many fluctuations in their feelings and behavior.[9]

Dental professionals may be involved with patients who are in any of these stages. An understanding of each person's expression of the stage of grief is essential for developing realistic dental treatment plans that are accepted by the patient.

Shock usually occurs during the acute phase of the injury. During this stage the patient feels completely overwhelmed, dependent, isolated, and confused. Although it is easy to identify and sympathize with the person's tragedy at this point, health care providers need to emphasize and demonstrate professional competence and expertise to foster a long-term, trusting relationship.

Once the initial shock has dissipated, the patient may assume an escapist attitude and deny certain aspects of the disability. A professional display of empathy rather than logical explanations are most helpful in enabling the patient to focus on daily realities and responsibilities. At some point the patient realizes the disability and reactions may include overt anger, depression, or withdrawal. Attempts to involve withdrawn or depressed patients in activities and provide positive situations to increase their confidence and self-image will facilitate re-entry into daily life activities. Angry patients are more difficult to handle, especially if they become physically aggressive. Professionals should not take the patient's actions personally or be judgmental. These patients need to have limits set as well as alternative methods for expressing their anger.

During the fourth stage of mobilization, the patient adjusts to reality and begins to participate in the rehabilitation process. The patient is now open to planning and problem-solving sessions, as well as learning new knowledge and skills. This period is generally the time to initiate new treatment regimens or suggestions. As the patient progresses through re-integration into community life, the fifth stage—coping—becomes a primary focus in dealing with activities of daily living.

TREATMENT AND REHABILITATION

Immediate hospital management of the person with spinal cord injury includes x-ray examination and neurologic examination to determine the location and extent of the injury and catheterization to allow the bladder to drain. In Europe most people with spinal cord injuries are transported to special spinal injury units within a day or two of injury. At present, about 15 such centers exist in the United States.[3,5,6,7,10]

Rehabilitation begins as soon as the diagnosis is made. The goals of initial treatment are to make the patient less dependent on any mechanical apparatus and to decrease the direct nursing care needs. Emotional and psychological needs are also a priority at this point. As rehabilitation continues through several months, four other areas of care in the program include: increasing specific skills through physical exercises; using equipment intended to replace lost muscle function and allow maximum independence; designing the living and working environment to adapt to the person's limitations, and providing vocational/educational training for living activities and regular follow-up.[10]

A team approach is used for managing the patient's problems and for developing unique programs for each individual's needs. Primary team members usually include physicians, nurses, counselors, and therapists (occupational, physical, speech, and recreational). Other health care providers, such as dental professionals, respiratory therapists, dieticians, and vocational specialists, may be called upon at periodic intervals. Dentists may be asked to fabricate mouth sticks for quadriplegics to use for turning pages, writing, drawing, typing, and other functions. The type of mouth stick fabricated depends on its intended use (Fig. 6–2).[11,12] As treatment and rehabilitation continue, movement and mobility are major problems that can be managed through exercise and adaptive equipment such as wheelchairs and braces. The degree of motor impairment depends upon the level of the injury. Spasticity, which consists of reflex-type movements that occur with intact reflex arcs

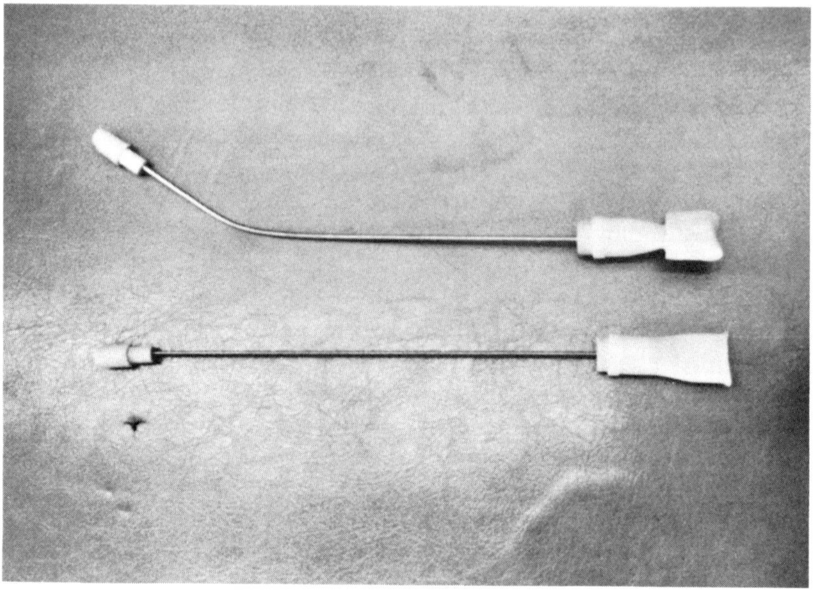

Fig. 6–2. Quadriplegics may have to depend on mouthsticks to aid them in accomplishment of daily tasks.

after spinal shock has subsided, can result in contractures. Contractures also occur early in treatment due to immobilization and tightness of the joints. Treatment for spasticity includes exercise, drug therapy, such as diazepam (Valium), dantrolene (Dantrium), or baclofen (Lioresal), and radio frequency rhizotomy, which destroys certain fibers in the sensory system. Bony accumulations called heterotopic ossifications may also develop around knee and hip joints.

Respiration may be compromised, particularly with cervical and upper thoracic injuries. Paralysis of the intercostal muscles creates dyspnea and requires diaphragmatic respiration. Tracheostomy is sometimes necessary, as well as mechanical ventilation during the acute stages postinjury or on a permanent basis for people with C1, C2, or C3 injuries. Oral reflexes such as coughing or gagging may also be diminished. Sensory systems below the site of injury are impaired and create safety problems because of the inability to perceive pain, pressure, and touch. Patients, however, may complain of "pain"; these sensations are not actually those of pain, but discomfort associated with healing or at junctional or distal sites from the injury. Acetaminophen (Tylenol) is generally prescribed for these sensations, since classic pain medications (narcotics) are not effective. Decubitus ulcers (pressure sores) develop easily when the patient remains in one position for prolonged periods; these can be avoided by frequent changes in position, appropriate padding, and support of the buttocks region.

The autonomic nervous system is usually affected, creating problems with bladder, bowel, and vasomotor control, as well as sexual function. Incomplete emptying of the bladder (neurogenic bladder) can lead to infection and calculi. Urinary problems such as kidney stones or inflammation are the main cause of death in patients with spinal cord injuries. Bladder problems are managed by the insertion of indwelling catheters. Male patients usually wear external urine collectors attached to the leg. Female patients are more prone to urinary infections and are given medications to prevent urine dribbling. Males who do not require catheters perform reflex voiding, but still usually wear external collectors. Antibiotics such as tetracycline, cephalexin (Keflex), or ampicillin and antibacterial agents such as Septra or nitrofurantoin (Macrodantin) may be prescribed. Anticholinergics such as oxyphencyclimine (Daricon) are also used.

The bowels are usually emptied at *regular* intervals (e.g., every morning) by taking advantage of an easily established reflex that causes the sphincter to relax and peristalsis to move the stool down the colon to the exterior. This reflex is initiated by means of a rectal suppository or digital stimulation. Dietary management and docusate (Dialose) and Metamucil are used as stool softeners. A colostomy (a surgically created opening through the abdominal wall for emptying fecal material) may have to be performed as a last resort.

Gastrointestinal problems also require dietary modifications. Patients are advised to avoid dairy products, potatoes, citrus fruits, and carbonated beverages. They are encouraged to eat vegetables and noncitrus fruits containing vitamin C. Liquid refreshment generally consists of cranberry, apple, and grape juice.

DENTAL MANAGEMENT

Acute

Since spinal cord injuries result from accidents, trauma to the face and jaws are the most common initial dental problems. Fractures and abrasions require prompt treatment in conjunction with the other conditions caused by the accident. Only dental professionals who work in hospital settings are involved with the dental management of these patients during this period. Patients may require surgical procedures that include immobilization of fractured jaws or facial reconstruction. The role of the dental auxiliary in this

TABLE 6–1. Task Analysis of Toothbrushing

1. Procure own toothbrush.
2. Approach sink, turn on water.
3. Wet toothbrush.
4. Remove toothpaste cap.
5. Spread paste on brush.
6. Grasp brush.
7. Place brush in mouth.
8. Brush all areas (list all areas).
9. Remove brush from mouth.
10. Spit out excess paste.
11. Rinse brush.
12. Rinse mouth.
13. Dry hands and mouth.
14. Store materials.

case would be to provide consultation and instruction to nursing staff for oral care procedures.

Intermediate

During the first few months of rehabilitation, most dental treatment usually has to be performed in a hospital or inpatient setting. Self-care skills for toothbrushing should be taught in conjunction with other personal hygiene skills. The dental hygienist or dental assistant may be asked to teach the patient directly or to develop a program to be implemented by others such as the occupational therapist. A task analysis of the steps involved in toothbrushing may be helpful for hospital staff as well as for analyzing problem areas and developing adaptations for these problems (Table 6–1).

Grasping the toothbrush can be a major problem for the person with a spinal cord injury. Paraplegics and persons with C7–C8 injuries generally experience no difficulties. Quadriplegics in the C5 and C6 classification do experience a variety of problems. Adaptive equipment is usually required for wrist stability, pincer grasp, and arm movements. Electric or manual toothbrushes and floss holders may be inserted into a universal cuff or a wrist-driven flexor-hinge hand brace (Figs. 6–3, 6–4). Angulation of the brush to reach all areas is occasionally an obstacle because of the lack of wrist rotation.

Manipulation of toothpaste is accomplished in a variety of ways. The toothpaste cap can be removed more easily by inserting a safety pin through the cap (Fig. 6–5). The tube can be held with both hands and squeezed, laid on a table and pressure applied, or squeezed with a plastic or metal roller. The paste can be applied directly into the mouth if the patient is unable to squeeze toothpaste onto the brush.

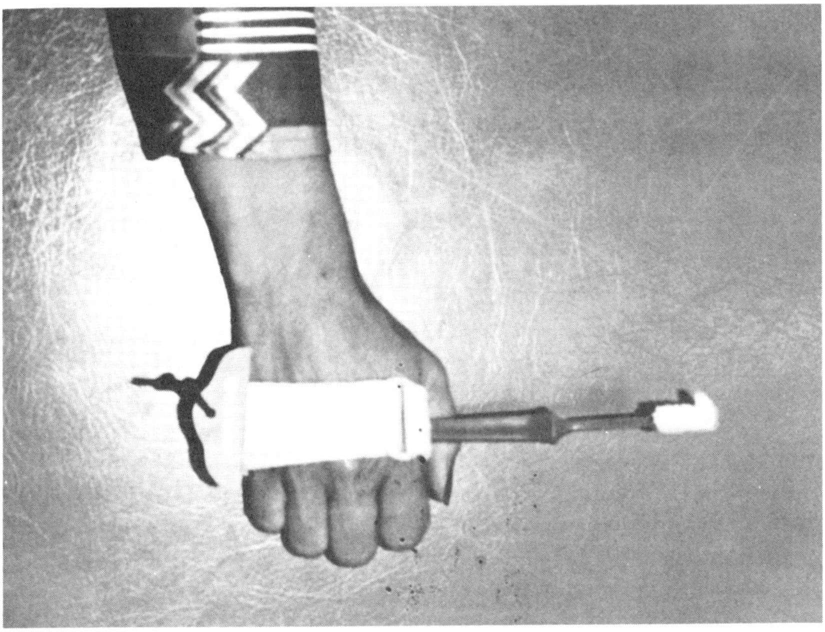

Fig. 6–3. A universal cuff can assist quadriplegics to maintain oral health.

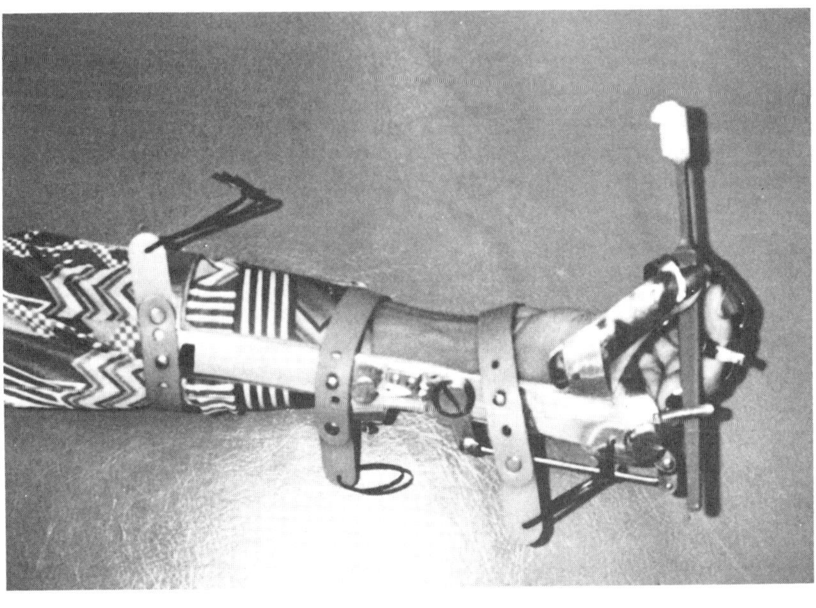

Fig. 6–4. Adaptive equipment can be used to aid in the maintenance of oral health.

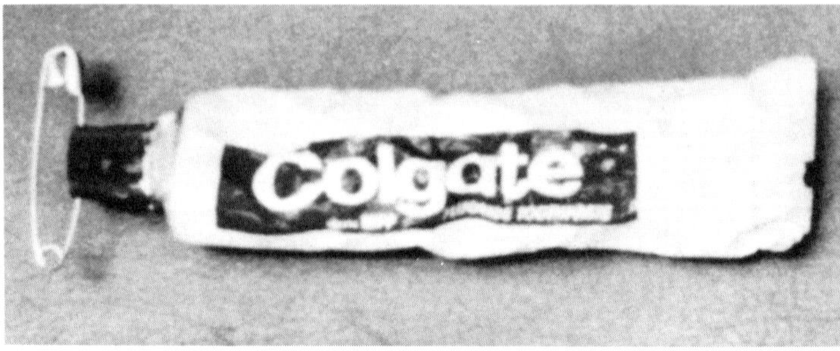

Fig. 6–5. A safety pin placed through the cap of a toothpaste tube allows easier access to toothpaste.

C1–C4 quadriplegics are totally dependent on others for oral hygiene care. Excessive amounts of foamy toothpaste should not be used since respiration is severely compromised and patients may depend on ventilators. Mouth sticks used by patients also require daily cleaning.

When designing oral hygiene programs, the patient's emotional status in relation to the five stages of grief is extremely important. Heroic efforts to teach self-care will not be successful until the patient is receptive to learning the skills and assuming the responsibility for self-care. Oral hygiene programs should also be based on the individual's existing oral conditions and identified risk factors for development of dental disease, such as the status of oral motor dysfunction, diet limitations, and general attitude.

Normalization

As rehabilitation progresses the patient resumes living in a community setting and will be ready to seek dental care. Access to the dental environment is the foremost environmental concern. If the dental office is not accessible or not relatively barrier-free, the wheelchair patient cannot obtain dental services. Curbs, stairs, narrow doors, thick carpeting, the size of the operatory, and dental chairs with nonadjustable or nonremovable arms can create barriers that are difficult to negotiate and may be insurmountable. Publications are available that can help a dental team evaluate the accessibility of the office.[13] As many barriers as possible should be adjusted or removed, or alternative patterns of access should be identified.

Another environmental factor under the control of the dental team is the regulation of temperatures in the waiting room and operatory. Since autonomic regulation is lost below the site of the injury, the body's ability to regulate body temperature is impaired.

In a cold room the affected body parts will lose heat; in a warm room the patient will not sweat, resulting in a rise in body temperature. To protect patients from gains and losses in body heat and to ensure comfort, room temperature should be carefully controlled.[7]

Wheelchair Transfer. The wheelchair can be an environmental barrier to dental treatment if the dental team is not familiar with the different types of wheelchairs. Considerations for moving patients depend on the dental diagnostic or treatment procedures being performed, the weight of the patient, the type of wheelchair, wheelchair attachments, and other factors such as medical problems. Head rests can be attached to the back of wheelchairs and used for examinations and selected treatments. An extension-type prosthetic headrest can be attached to a dental chair and rotated 180° so that a wheelchair can be backed up to the dental chair.[14] Patients who need to be transferred to the dental chair generally prefer to transfer themselves or be assisted by an accompanying friend or relative. If dental team members have to provide assistance, the patient should be asked to explain the preferred method of transfer and any necessary precautions. A patient may wish to use a transfer board (Fig. 6–6) of his or her own, or the dental office may wish to purchase or construct one. Before any transfer, make sure that the rear wheels on the wheelchair are in the locked position and front wheels are locked forward. Also, have the patient check any urinary catheters or leg bags before and after transfer.

PREVENTIVE MEASURES

Problems that may impact on dental treatment include prevention of decubitus ulcers, dealing with muscle spasticity, respiratory impairment, medication regimens, orthopedic braces, and impaired bladder and bowel control. Most patients will not be sitting in a dental chair for prolonged periods of time, but frequent opportunities for shifting weight should be provided to prevent pressure on sensitive areas. Orthopedic braces can interfere with patient comfort in contoured dental chairs. Removal of the braces may be advisable during dental treatment (Fig. 6–7). Uncontrollable muscle spasticity may occur periodically and interfere with treatment. Procedures should be discontinued momentarily until the muscle activity subsides.

Patients may ask for assistance with special techniques for coughing. Adequate suction and airway protection is extremely important. Determination of a comfortable chair position for the patient depends on the level of injury and the degree of respiratory impairment. Patients should be asked which position they prefer. Patients

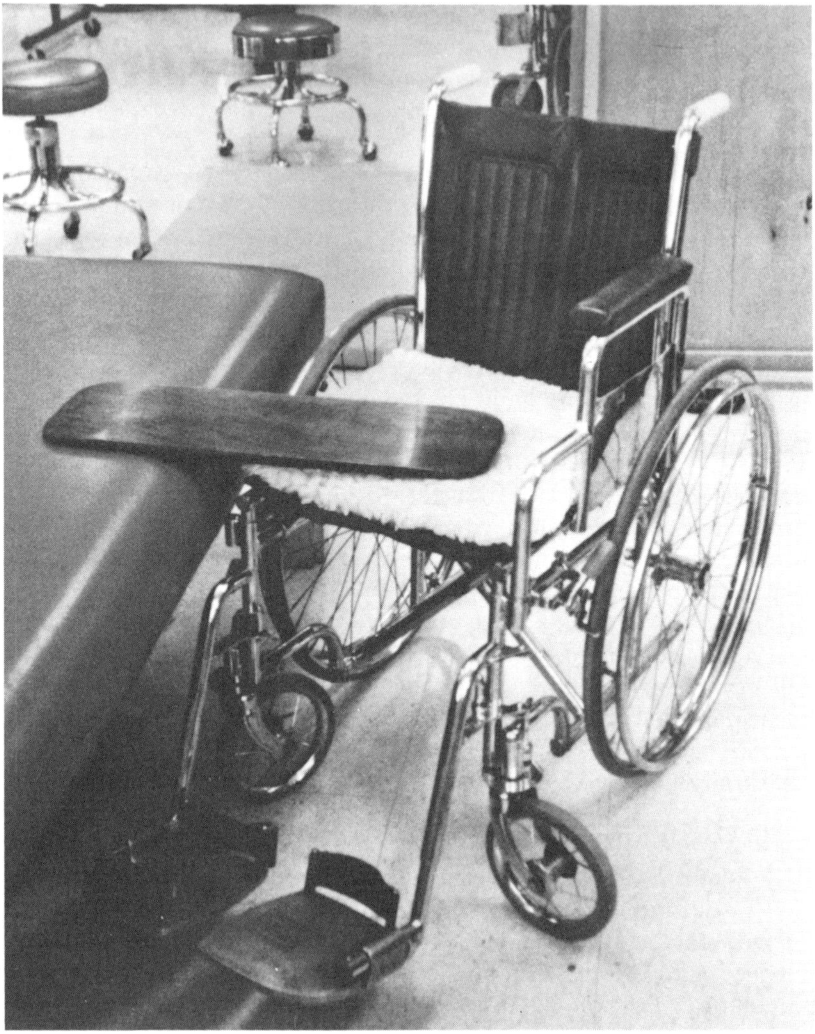

Fig. 6–6. The use of a transfer board allows the patient to maintain a sense of independence.

may be taking multiple medications, therefore a physician's consultation is indicated to avoid possible dental-related drug interactions.

TREATMENT PLANNING

Treatment planning options may be dictated by the level of spinal injury and the degree to which the patient uses his or her mouth for various purposes. The mouth and the teeth play a vital

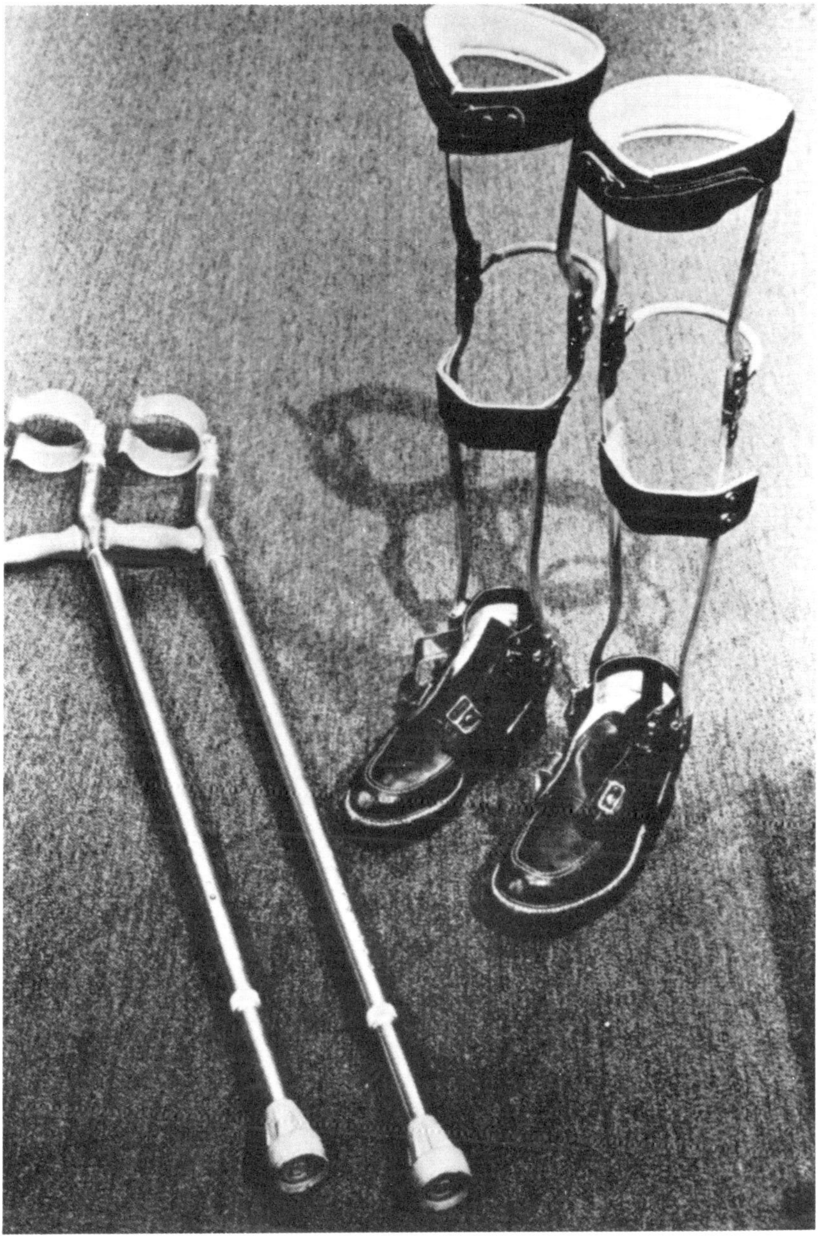

Fig. 6–7. Leg braces can prevent a patient from getting comfortable. Leg braces also damage a dental chair if proper precautions are not taken. (Photo of the Scott-Craig long leg brace reproduced from Functional Goals at Specific Levels of Spinal Cord Injury, by permission of M. Greb, J.M. Mueller.)

role in grasping, stabilizing, and opening objects to compensate for loss of hand and arm function. A phenomenal degree of stress is therefore placed on the teeth. Removable dental appliances are probably not feasible in these instances.

Edentulous quadriplegic patients are considered severely handicapped because of the problems they have in using mouth sticks. Cleaning the mouthpiece portion of the stick can be incorporated into the daily oral hygiene routine of brushing and rinsing.[15] Mouth sticks also place a great deal of stress on the oral structures and cause extensive attrition of teeth. Dental professionals play a vital role in convincing patients with spinal cord injuries of the importance of maintaining dental health and contribute to the support of optimal independence for the individual.

PATIENT SCENARIOS

Situation 1

Description

You have been asked by a spinal injury center to develop a preventive dental program for approximately 40 patients who participate in an extensive rehabilitation program for six months. These patients have a variety of spinal injuries and individual needs.

Anticipated Needs

—information about types of injuries
—teaching aids
—a variety of adapted toothbrushes

Awareness Strategies

1. How will you approach instruction for 40 patients with individualized needs?
2. What supplies will you request?
3. How will you schedule your teaching program?
4. What method of follow-up will you implement?

Situation 2

Description

You have been asked to develop a table clinic on dental office management of patients with spinal injuries who are now reintegrated into the community.

Anticipated Needs

—a selected topic for presentation
—visual aids
—development of ten-minute narration

Awareness Strategies

1. Which topic would be most suitable for table clinic presentation?
2. What kinds of information would be most beneficial to your audience?
3. What examples of aids could you use in preparing your presentation?
4. How can you assure transfer of information to your audience?

Patient 1

Description

Bob M. is a 33-year-old paraplegic who is scheduled for an office visit for the first time.

Anticipated Needs

—evaluation of barriers
—status of oral health
—status of physical capabilities
—treatment planning

Awareness Strategies

1. What steps will you take prior to Bob's arrival in the office?
2. How will you prepare to accommodate Bob's dental examination?
3. What information do you need to complete Bob's medical and dental history?
4. How will you plan for Bob's home care needs?

REFERENCES

1. Gutterman, L.: Spinal Cord Injuries. Oxford, Blackwell Scientific Publications, 1976.
2. Bromley, I.: Tetraplegia and Paraplegia. Edinburgh, Churchill Livingstone, 1981.
3. Sutton, N.: Injuries of the Spinal Cord: The Management of Paraplegia and Tetraplegia. London, Butterworths, 1973.
4. Adams, R., Daniel, A., McCubbin, J., and Rullman, L.: Games, Sports and Exercises for the Physically Handicapped. ed. 2. Philadelphia, Lea & Febiger, 1982.
5. U.S. Department of Health, Education and Welfare: Spinal Cord Injury: Hope

Through Research. Public Health Service Publication No. 1747, Health Information Series No. 143, Washington, D.C., 1968.
6. Nagel, D.: Traumatic paraplegia and quadriplegia. *In* Physically Handicapped Children: A Medical Atlas for Teachers. Edited by E.E. Bleck and D.A. Nagel. New York, Grune & Stratton, 1975.
7. Krengel, J.R., and Rohrer, L.M.: Paraplegic and Quadriplegic Individuals. Chicago, The National Paraplegia Foundation, 1977.
8. Bedbrook, G.: The Care and Management of Spinal Cord Injuries. New York, Springer Verlag, 1981.
9. Manley, S.: Five Stages of Grief. Handout No. 8520, Craig Hospital, Denver, CO, June, 1979.
10. Craig Hospital: The Spinal Injury Program. Englewood, CO, Rocky Mountain Regional Spinal Injury Center, Inc.
11. Donnelly, M., and Beder, O.: A manipulative appliance. J. Prosthet. Dent., *28*:309–312, 1972.
12. Baline, H., and Nelson, E.: A mouthstick for quadriplegic patients. J. Prosthet. Dent., *29*:317–322, 1973.
13. Illustrated Standards for Public Buildings. 1975. The Public Buildings Safety Committee, State Building Division, D.A.S., State Capitol Building, Lincoln, NE 68509.
14. McGhay, R.M.: Simple headrest for patients confined to wheelchairs. J. Prosthet. Dent. *44*:347–349, 1980.
15. Durnan, R., and Thaler, R.: Dental care for the patient with a spinal cord injury. Journal of the American Dental Association, JADA, *86*:1318–1321, 1973.

Chapter 7

MULTIPLE SCLEROSIS

Imagine becoming aware of a tingling sensation in your legs that seems to come and go and you cannot determine its cause. After a week or so, the sensation lasts longer, and at times, one or both legs feel as though they are asleep. When you decide to go to the doctor the symptoms disappear, and you think nothing more about them until they reappear six months later. This time the symptoms of tingling and numbness are in your hands and arms as well as your feet and legs. You make an appointment to see your doctor; he can find nothing wrong with you. Yet the numbness spreads. Your eye-hand coordination is also becoming impaired. You are hospitalized and given thorough examinations including x-rays, an upper and lower G.I. series, and a spinal tap, but no cause for your symptoms is determined. At this point the discomfort of the examinations, the worry about your physical health and the cost of the procedures, and the concern of your family begin to overwhelm you.

The foregoing sequence of events is experienced by many individuals each year. The time intervals and symptoms vary, but the mental and emotional stress of multiple sclerosis are perhaps the most devastating of any of the handicapping conditions. Young adults with this condition experience great anxiety from the worsening physical condition, the lack of a specific diagnosis and treatment plan, and the unexpected interruptions in their lives and careers.

DEFINITION

Multiple sclerosis is described as a chronic degenerative disease of the central nervous system.[1] Classified as a "demyelinating disease," it affects the myelin or white matter of the brain and spinal cord. Myelin is a fatty substance that surrounds and insulates each

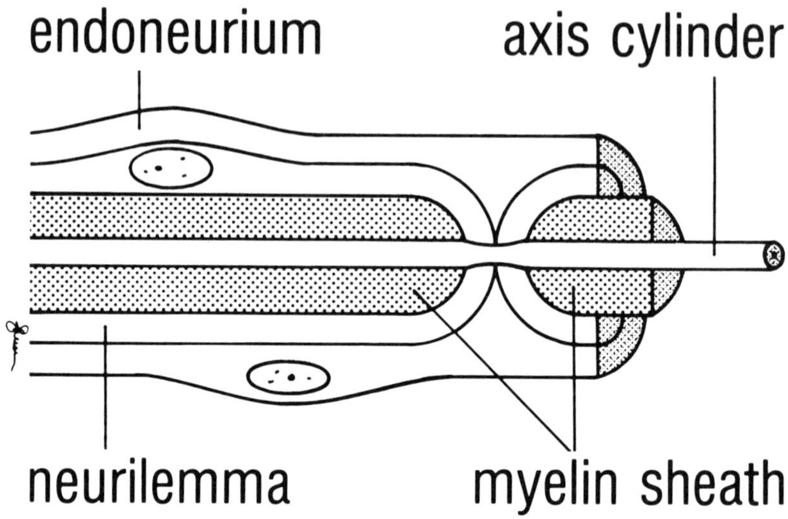

Fig. 7–1. The structure of a normal nerve fiber.

nerve fiber of the central nervous system (Fig. 7–1). Patches or sections of the myelin are destroyed through the formation of sclerotic tissue called plaque. As the plaque replaces the myelin, the nerve fibers begin to degenerate. The accumulation of plaque continues until the nerve becomes permanently damaged or destroyed. Consequently, nerve impulses to the brain become disrupted or are not transmitted.[2–4] Plaque accumulation does not follow a pattern or sequence; consequently myelin destruction occurs in scattered areas, causing widespread and varied symptoms. The disease process tends to follow a cycle of exacerbation and remission, with each successive attack becoming more debilitating than the previous one.[1]

INCIDENCE AND ONSET

Approximately 500,000 people in the United States are believed to have multiple sclerosis. The incidence rate varies dramatically across the country. For example, the incidence rate in northern states is high (40 to 64 per 100,000), while in southern states it is as low as 7 to 15 per 100,000. Historically, researchers believed the incidence rate also varied across cultures. Kurouiva suggests that lower incidence rates in different societies are primarily a reflection of underdiagnosis, since many of these societies are in developing countries with shortages of medical personnel and facilities.[5] Nonetheless, a variance in incidence does exist in both developed and developing countries.

The incidence rate also varies with sex; women appear to have a higher incidence than men. A study by Leibowitz and Alter of multiple sclerosis patients in Israel revealed a female/male ratio of 1.08:1, with a higher ratio (1.5:1) at younger ages and a lower ratio (.95:1) for individuals over the age of forty.[6]

Multiple sclerosis occurs within extended families at a rate 5 to 20 times higher than that observed in the general population. Field cites genetic research that identified individuals at risk for developing multiple sclerosis.[7] All of those identified as being at high risk, however, did not develop the disease.

The onset of multiple sclerosis can occur at any age. The disease process is most commonly observed in persons between the ages of 20 and 45, with 30 being the modal age of onset. Researchers have not yet been able to explain the observed differences in terms of age, sex, predilection, or geography.[4,7]

ETIOLOGY

The cause of multiple sclerosis is unknown, although several theories are currently being postulated. Researchers are examining the role of infections, slow-acting viruses, antibody reactions in the central nervous system, deficiencies of essential fatty acids, and genetic defects as factors that contribute to the breakdown of myelin.[6,8]

One theory is that the plaque and resultant scars are precipitated by an autoimmune (allergic) reaction (antibrain antibodies attacking myelin) that occurs in the tiny capillaries of the blood-brain barrier where they anastomose to form veins.[3]

Another researcher suggests that multiple sclerosis is an interaction of genotype and environment, in which a "factor X" acts on susceptible genotypes.[7] Based on this theory, a genetic deficiency interferes with the production of essential fatty acids for myelination in the developmental period of life. The resultant lack of fatty acids leads to the production of substandard myelin. As the individual matures and is physiologically stressed by "factor X" (e.g., virus, allergy, or a high-fat diet), the myelin begins to break down. These theories lack sufficient supportive data at this time to provide an accepted explanation of the disease process of multiple sclerosis.

SYMPTOMS

Symptoms result from lesions caused by the breakdown of myelin or plaque in the central nervous system; they vary depending on the location of the lesions. The lesions occur in the spinal cord, brainstem, or cerebrum. Table 7–1 describes the symptoms according to these locations. Typically the symptoms are progressive. In the early stages of the disease, symptoms may resemble fatigue,

TABLE 7–1. Symptoms Associated with Lesions in the Central Nervous System.

Location of Lesions	Possible Symptoms
Spinal cord	Numbness Loss of sensitivity in appendages Sensitivity to heat Unsteady gait Loss of strength in the legs Impaired eye-hand coordination resulting in difficulty in fine motor movements
Brain stem	Blurred and/or double vision Difficulty in swallowing or chewing Diminished gag reflex Slurred speech
Cerebrum (lesions in the cerebrum usually occur in the latter stages of the disease process)	Disruptions in thinking Euphoria Depression Disruptions in behavior

so that a disease process may not be suspected. As the disease progresses, paralysis of the limbs may develop. In advanced cases, loss of bladder and bowel control may occur. Sexual impotence may also occur.

Multiple sclerosis is unique because the symptoms tend to improve (go into remission) regardless of treatment. Exacerbation of the disease process, particularly in the early stages of the disease, is thought to be triggered by such factors as fatigue, infections, pregnancy, or mental stress.[3]

DIAGNOSIS

The diagnosis of multiple sclerosis is a difficult task due to the variability of the symptoms. Diagnosis becomes more difficult if the primary demyelinating process occurs in the brain and the symptoms parallel other disorders.[6]

Currently, the diagnostic procedure used for any individual suspected of having multiple sclerosis reflects the training of the physician conducting the investigation. A diagnosis of multiple sclerosis is based primarily on the history of the lesion spread, the characteristic exacerbations and remissions, the geographic spread of the lesions, and the results of laboratory findings. Research continues towards developing and refining the diagnostic procedures. The various approaches include revising the criteria for diagnosis according to certain clinical and laboratory findings,[8,9] electrophysiologic tests,[10] or laboratory tests that identify how a person's body handles certain fatty acids.[7]

TREATMENT

Presently, multiple sclerosis cannot be cured. As with diagnostic techniques, the treatment used reflects the training of the physician or the theoretic approach supported by the researcher. Studies currently being carried out with interferon, a virus-blocking protein, show some promise in the treatment of multiple sclerosis.

Many physicians prescribe medication to relieve such symptoms as spasticity or visual disturbances. The use of adrenocortical stimulating hormone (ACTH) has proved beneficial in controlling exacerbations. However, prolonged use of the medication may have undesirable side effects.[7] Corticosteroids (prednisone) have also been used to reduce the severity of exacerbation. Patients may receive other medications for muscle spasms, pain, infections, and bladder problems.

Some physicians recommend a program of rest and exercise. Specifically, patients are advised to engage in short periods of strenuous exercise designed to improve circulation, followed by the exercising of specific body parts to maintain strength and coordination. Patients are also advised to lie down and rest for a few minutes at six-hour intervals.[3] Physical and occupational therapy may be useful for maintaining the strength and function of unaffected muscles and for assisting the patient in making adaptations for activities of daily living.

Field states that the breakdown in myelin can be controlled through a diet low in saturated (animal) fats and high in unsaturated (vegetable) fats. The mechanism behind the diet's reported effectiveness is not well understood.[7]

All treatment strategies are followed over a long period of time to study the effects of treatment during periods of exacerbation and remission. Often, researchers have been encouraged by a specific treatment only to discover that the disease was moving into a state of remission. Patients are usually instructed to avoid mental stress and physical fatigue, since these factors are recognized as contributing to the exacerbation of the disease process.

PSYCHOSOCIAL IMPLICATIONS

By the time a diagnosis of multiple sclerosis has been made, the affected patient has suffered great anxiety and stress, which in all likelihood intensified the symptoms. Because of the varying symptoms and often late diagnosis, many patients begin to question their own judgment, and in some cases their judgment is questioned by their family and physician. After the diagnosis is made, individuals may face a change in career plans and personal goals. They are also faced with a progressive disease that may slowly rob them of their motor abilities, eye-hand coordination, bladder and bowel control, and a potential decline in activities with family and friends.[1] Individual and family counseling may be helpful, in addition to participation in self-help groups.

The problems incurred in reaching a diagnosis, the adjustments made in life style, the mental stress of knowing the disease will progress, the loss of self-esteem that comes from these factors, and decreased contacts with friends can easily lead to changes in personality.[11] Reactions include denial, hostility, and withdrawal. When the cerebrum is affected by the disease, a person's thinking process and behavior may become abnormal. Caution should be exercised in assuming that a person with multiple sclerosis will have any of these personality reactions, since most are not manifested until late in the disease process, or may not be manifested at all. Dental team members should be aware of the stresses involved and the adjustments required in the life style of a person who has multiple sclerosis, and should adjust their expectations of patient behavior accordingly.

ORAL MANIFESTATIONS

No dental disease states are specifically inherent to multiple sclerosis. Any increased incidence of dental caries is probably attributable to poor oral hygiene, poor nutrition, or xerostomia caused by the medications. In the latter stage of the disease, oral hygiene care may be compromised by the patient's double vision, muscle weakness, tremors, reliance on other people for care, apathy, stress, or fatigue.

Little is mentioned in the dental literature of oral conditions specific to multiple sclerosis. Patients with persistent pain are often placed on carbamazepine (Tegretol) or phenytoin (Dilantin). Oral complications such as ulceration, xerostomia, or gingival overgrowth might accompany these drugs. If a patient with multiple sclerosis complains of facial pain, differential determination of the etiology of the pain is essential, since advanced dental caries and periodontal disease create similar pain sensations.

DENTAL MANAGEMENT

Many dental management considerations depend on the status of the disease at the time of the patient's appointment and the individual's reaction to the disease. Some patients with multiple sclerosis may show minimal symptoms and do not require any special management considerations. A patient who is newly diagnosed may be extremely depressed or overwhelmed by his or her situation and

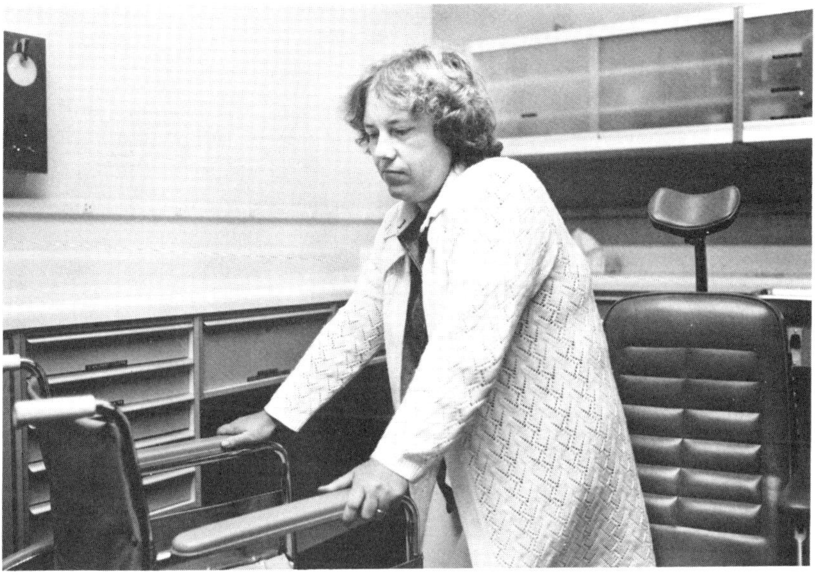

Fig. 7–2. Allow the patient to direct how he or she will be transferred from the wheelchair to the dental chair.

may refuse dental care, miss appointments, or be embarrassed to tell you of the disease. The task of dental team members is to convey empathy and concern in this situation, assuring the patient that the quality of dental care will not be compromised by the disease. The patient should be informed of the role infection plays in exacerbating the disease process, stressing the need for optimal oral hygiene and regular dental visits. Reinforcement of the patient's self-esteem is essential.

In any stage of the disease, allow enough time during appointments for the patient to talk about the disease, if he or she so desires. A complete medical history with constant updating will be necessary to record changes in symptoms, treatment regimens (including medications), and the patient's emotional status. Anecdotal notes can be useful for gathering this information. These factors are important for treatment planning, particularly as they affect the use of dentally related drugs. The administration of oral sedatives for the anxious patient will have to be weighed in terms of the potential interactions or depressant effects with medications being taken by the patient. If the patient fatigues easily, the appointment schedule may have to be adjusted to avoid undue stress.

A patient in the advanced stages of the disease may be wearing a catheter for bladder dysfunction and may need to empty the collecting bag, which can cause embarrassment if it interrupts the dental procedures. Embarrassment can be avoided by indicating to the patient the location of the restroom prior to dental treatment.

If the patient is confined to a wheelchair, the hallway and operatory should be cleared of obstacles that would prevent access, before summoning the patient. Once in the operatory, the patient's usual method of transfer from the wheelchair should be followed (Fig. 7–2), according to the guidelines for wheelchair transfers in Chapter 6. If the patient is catheterized, care should be taken to prevent applying pressure to the bag, thus avoiding leakage during transfer or when the patient is being positioned in the dental chair.

If the patient has difficulty in swallowing or a diminished gag reflex is evident, the patient's position should be adjusted to one that least compromises swallowing. The use of a rubber dam is indicated for restorative procedures, and frequent mouth evacuation is essential. Periodic reassurance will reduce the patient's anxiety in this situation. Muscle weakness may limit the length of time the patient can maintain an open mouth; the use of a mouth prop may facilitate operator access, reduce patient fatigue, and help the patient to compensate for weakness. Progressive weakness of the facial and masticatory muscles may interfere with proper denture fit in edentulous patients, necessitating more frequent visits for adjustment.

Treatment planning for the multiple sclerosis patient should include alternative provisions for treatment in the event of financial difficulties or extended periods of disease exacerbation. Assistance in developing a personalized home care program should be provided along with preventive procedures.

PREVENTIVE MEASURES

Home care recommendations are determined by certain factors:

1. Patient's attitudes toward preventive care
2. Emotional status
3. Motor coordination
4. Nutritional status

Usually these factors act in combination rather than singly. Patients who exhibit poor nutritional states may have lost their appetite, may have developed poor habits as a result of stress and depression, or may have impaired utilization of nutrients (a possible side effect of medications). It is important to use a comprehensive approach in assessing preventive needs and the patient's potential for complying with recommendations.

Motor coordination problems, tremors, and muscle weakness should also be assessed carefully to determine the degree to which they affect both in-office and home care procedures. The patient's stability problems can usually be overcome in the office by the use of mouth props and effective head and jaw control by the dental staff. This situation demands adaptations made by the dental staff, not by the patient. Home care procedures, on the other hand, require the patient's cooperation and evaluation to be successful. Toothbrushing instructions should take into account the person's hand strength, fatigue factor, and ability to place the brush on the teeth and produce a brushing stroke; the positioning of the patient and the availability of others to assist are also important. Modifications should be suggested as necessary. For instance, grasping a regular toothbrush with two hands may be easier for the patient than supporting the weight and controlling the movements of an electric brush. Tremors might be controlled by supporting the elbows and head during oral care procedures. Recommendations for substantial assistance by another person may be made after consultation with the patient. The goal of all adaptations for home care is to provide effective, acceptable methods for oral hygiene maintenance that promote the highest level of independent functioning by the patient.

PATIENT SCENARIOS

Patient 1

Description

Mrs. T. is 28 years old, married, and a regular patient in your office. When you call to schedule a recall appointment, her husband informs you that she has recently been diagnosed as having multiple sclerosis. She has been depressed but will come in for her appointment.

Anticipated Needs

—updated health history
—recall examination and prophylaxis
—home care instructions

Awareness Strategies

1. How can you make Mrs. T. feel at ease in the office?
2. What questions should you ask her about her newly diagnosed condition?
3. Are there any oral conditions that you should inform Mrs.

T. about that are related to multiple sclerosis?
4. What symptoms might she exhibit while in the dental chair?

Patient 2

Description

Mr. S. is a 50-year-old college professor who calls your office complaining of facial pain. He states that he has multiple sclerosis and is confined to a wheelchair. He transports himself in his van. He is concerned about missing his lectures.

Anticipated Needs

—comprehensive examination
—x-rays
—possible treatment
—another appointment
—home care instructions

Awareness Strategies

1. What information should you gather over the telephone to prepare for Mr. S's appointment?
2. How can you assist him in transferring from the wheelchair?
3. What precautions will you take if Mr. S. has bladder problems?
4. What problems do you anticipate in providing home care instructions?

REFERENCES

1. Davis, M.Z.: Living with Multiple Sclerosis: A Social Psychological Analysis. Springfield, Ill., Charles C Thomas, 1973.
2. Guyton, A.G.: Textbook of Medical Physiology. Philadelphia, W.B. Saunders Co., 1976.
3. Russell, W.: Multiple Sclerosis: Control of the Disease. New York, Pergamon Press, 1976.
4. Robbins, S.L.: Pathology. ed. 3. Philadelphia, W.B. Saunders, 1967.
5. Kurouiva, Y.: Multiple Sclerosis in Asia. Baltimore, University Park Press, 1975.
6. Leibowitz, U., and Alter, M.: Multiple Sclerosis: Clues to Its Cause. New York, North-Holland Publishing Co., 1973.
7. Field, E.J.: Multiple Sclerosis in Childhood. Springfield, Ill., Charles C Thomas, 1980.
8. Maugh, T.H.: Multiple sclerosis: two or more viruses may be involved. Science, *195*:768–771, 1977.
9. Bauer, H.J.: IMAB-Enquête concerning the diagnostic criteria for M.S. *In* Progress in Multiple Sclerosis Research. Edited by H.J. Bauer, S. Poser, and G. Ritter. New York, Springer-Verlag, 1980.
10. McDonald, W.I.: The role of evoked potentials in the diagnosis of multiple sclerosis. *In* Progress in Multiple Sclerosis Research. Edited by H.J. Bauer, S. Poser, and G. Ritter. New York, Springer-Verlag, 1980.
11. Herbold, E., and Lindenmuth, J.: Communication in patient management as seen in a patient with multiple sclerosis. JADA, 97:487–488, 1979.

Chapter 8
MUSCULAR DYSTROPHY

. . . He had accepted his problem. He learned to live not walking, And found his soul had wings to fly above the earth.[1]

Such are the thoughts of a young poet who campaigned for the rights of handicapped persons and died at the age of 21 of Duchenne's muscular dystrophy. Although not always fatal, the muscular dystrophies comprise a large portion of childhood muscular disorders. Dental professionals should be prepared to manage patients with any degree of impairment caused by these crippling diseases in a setting that is least traumatic and stressful for the patient.

DEFINITION

The term muscular dystrophy is used to identify a group of progressive chronic diseases of the skeletal (striated) muscles. The disease process is characterized by a systematic degeneration of muscle cells that starts with atrophy; after sufficient musculature has atrophied, deformity begins to occur. If the deformity is severe enough, disability is the result. The sequence of degeneration is the same for all forms of muscular dystrophy; only the age of onset and rate of progression vary. The degeneration begins with a swelling of the affected muscle cells, followed by the breaking up of the bands across the muscles. The cytoplasm then becomes homogeneous in appearance, and finally, fat deposits replace the muscle tissue (Fig. 8–1). As affected muscles break down, healthy muscle tissue begins to compensate, causing added stress and muscle pseudohypertrophy.[2–4]

INCIDENCE AND CLASSIFICATION

Approximately 150,000 to 200,000 people in the United States have some form of muscular dystrophy. The Duchenne, limb-

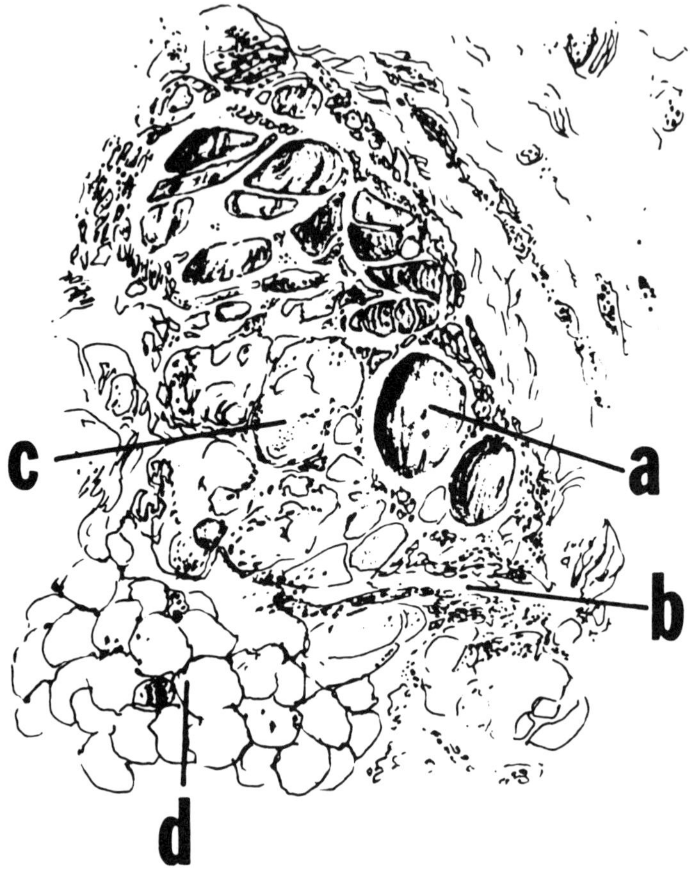

a. swelling of muscle cells
b. breaking of bands
c. cytoplasm
d. fat deposits

Fig. 8–1. The process of degeneration of striated muscle.

girdle, and fascioscapulohumeral forms of muscular dystrophy are the three most commonly observed and the best defined. More than half of those affected are children between the ages of 4 and 15. The Duchenne type is the most commonly observed form, affecting about 270 out of every 1,000,000 live male births. The limb-

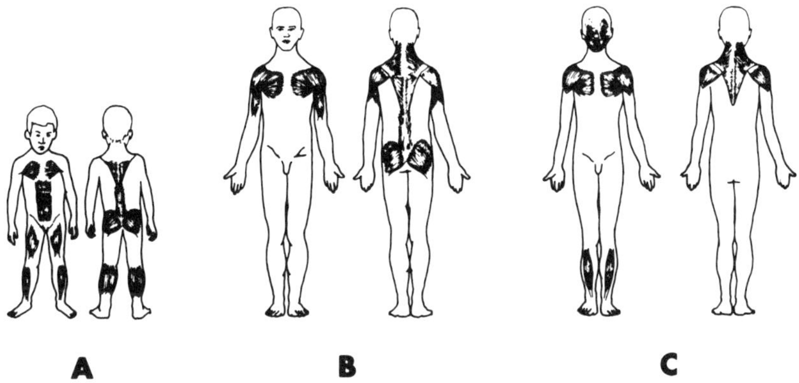

Fig. 8–2. Early distribution of muscle weakness in the three major forms of muscular dystrophy: (A) Duchenne's dystrophy; (B) limb girdle dystrophy; (C) fascioscapulohumeral dystrophy. Reproduced by permission from I.M. Siegel.

girdle form affects 65 out of every 1,000,000 live births; the fascioscapulohumeral type, 4 per 1,000,000. Other forms are rather uncommon.[3,5,6]

Each form has different symptoms and an identifiable sequence of progression. Classification depends largely on the age of the patient at onset, the muscles affected, the hereditary pattern, and the clinical course (Fig. 8–2).

SYMPTOMS AND ETIOLOGY

Duchenne's Muscular Dystrophy

Duchenne's muscular dystrophy mainly affects boys and is the most destructive and progressive of all the types (Fig. 8–3). The symptoms usually become evident around age three, when the loss of a third or more of the muscle tissue impairs muscle function. Typically, within a few years of diagnosis, the individual becomes debilitated and confined to bed. Symptoms generally include clumsiness, with frequent falls and fractures, toe-walking, lordosis (waddling gait), cramping of the legs and abdomen, Gower's sign or "tripoding" (Fig. 8–4), inability to jump from the standing position, and decreased stamina.[3,5] The muscles of the pelvis, abdomen, hip and spine are affected first. Atrophy and weakness generally spread to the trunk and then to all extremities. The myocardium is also affected and changes to scar tissue. Cranial nerves are generally normal and sensation is not affected. Several radiographic findings, such as osteoporosis, are also noted.

Complications may occur once the person is confined to a wheelchair. These include:

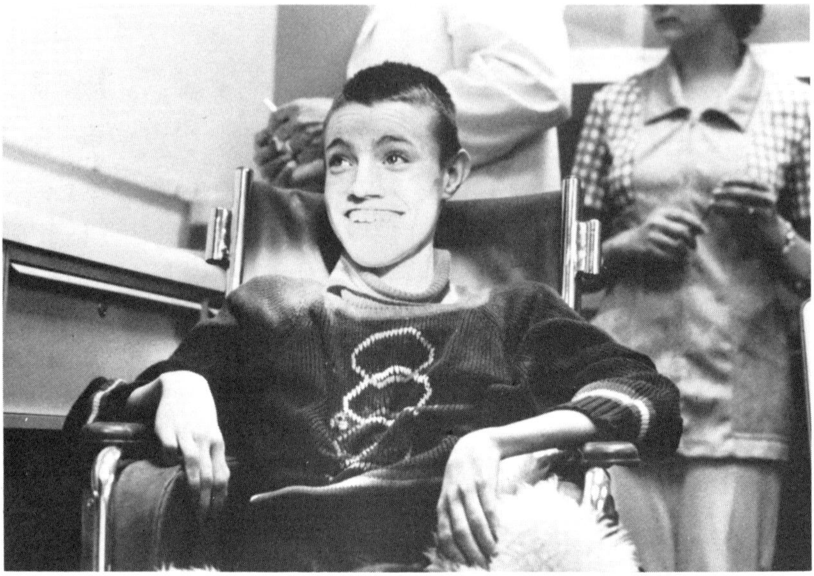

Fig. 8–3. Advanced stage of Duchenne's muscular dystrophy.

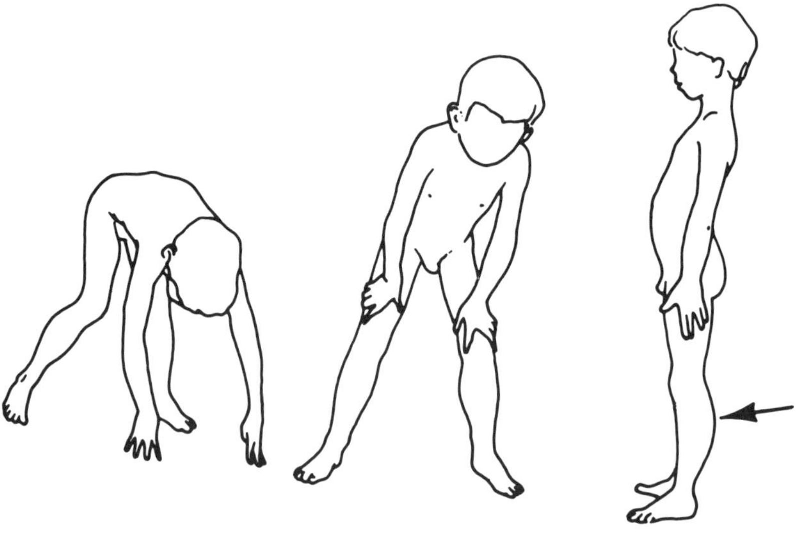

Fig. 8–4. Gower's sign. The child gets up from the floor by walking up his thighs with his hands due to weakness of the thigh muscles. The arrow points to the enlarged calves (pseudohypertrophy). (Reproduced by permission from Bleck, E.E.: Muscular dystrophy, Duchenne type. *In* Physically Handicapped Children: A Medical Atlas for Teachers. Edited by E.E. Bleck and D.A. Nagel. New York, Grune & Stratton, 1975.)

1. Scoliosis
2. Obesity
3. Increased cardiopulmonary problems
4. Decreased metabolic rate
5. Decreased circulation to extremities, with resultant edema
6. Increased atrophy, weakness, and joint contractures

These complications affect activities of daily living and require extensive time, effort, and understanding.[3] Death usually occurs in the midteens as a result of respiratory infection or respiratory failure. Cardiac problems include dyspnea, fatigue, tachycardia, and congestive heart failure, but rarely do they cause death.

Duchenne muscular dystrophy is a genetic disorder—specifically, a sex-linked recessive trait with a high mutation rate. Approximately one-third of the cases are sporadic mutations. The risk for transmission is 50% for sons of carrier mothers. One-half of the daughters of carrier women are carriers. The female carriers most often are symptom-free, but may exhibit a mild form of the degenerative process, which progresses at a slower rate.[7]

Beiker type X-linked muscular dystrophy is a variety that has a distribution of muscle weakness and genetic transmission similar to Duchenne muscular dystrophy. The Beiker type usually has a later onset and runs a milder course, with many individuals not experiencing symptoms until adult life. Individual cases may be difficult to distinguish from the more progressive Duchenne type.[8,9]

Limb-Girdle Dystrophy

The onset of the limb-girdle (Erb) form of muscular dystrophy occurs between the first and fifth decades of life, with the majority of individuals diagnosed in their second decade. The progression of limb-girdle dystrophy is slower than the Duchenne form; however, in some cases, progression can be rapid with loss of ambulation within three to four years after diagnosis. Many individuals with limb-girdle dystrophy are severely disabled by midlife and have a shorter life span than their peers. Typically, initial weakness occurs in the pelvic girdle, followed by weakness in the shoulder girdle. Onset is gradual, progressing from pain in affected muscles after exercise to total involvement of the muscle. The prognosis is better if weakness first appears in the shoulder girdle.[3,5,8,10] Limb-girdle dystrophy is inherited through an autosomal recessive pattern (both parents carry the affected gene). Consequently, both male and female offspring of parents who are carriers have a 25% chance of being affected and a 50% chance of being carriers.[8,10]

Fascioscapulohumeral Muscular Dystrophy

Fascioscapulohumeral muscular dystrophy is less frequently seen than the Duchenne and the limb-girdle forms. It is also the least destructive and progresses most slowly. Onset usually occurs at puberty, but may occur as late as the fourth decade. The disease may remain in a state of indefinite remission, with some individuals living a symptom-free, normal life span. Typically, the facial muscles are affected first, with the person encountering difficulty in wrinkling the forehead, puffing the cheeks, and fully closing the eyelids and lips. Weakness is primarily asymmetrical in distribution and degree. Over a period of time the person with fascioscapulohumeral dystrophy develops masklike, wrinklefree, expressionless facial features.

As the disease progresses, involvement of the shoulder girdle and upper arm becomes evident. Typically, muscles above the elbow atrophy, while muscles below the elbow remain intact. (The resultant effect is best illustrated by the arms of the cartoon character, Popeye.) The pelvic girdle muscles may also be affected; however, this type of muscle involvement varies greatly. Fascioscapulohumeral dystrophy is generally transmitted as an autosomal dominant trait (one parent has the gene; there is no carrier state), but in rare cases it may be a recessive gene. When one parent has fascioscapulohumeral dystrophy, each child has a 50% chance of being affected.[8,10]

The defect in all dystrophies is thought to be biochemical. Researchers have been unable to discover the cause(s) of the defect, and therefore, the etiology remains unknown.

DIAGNOSIS

Many children are misdiagnosed early and may see numerous specialists before a definitive diagnosis is made. Symptoms are sometimes confused with those of other muscular diseases, metabolic disorders, or neuropathies. Diagnosis is based on a clinical history, familial genetic workup, physical examination, and laboratory tests. Laboratory tests include analysis of red blood cells and muscle enzymes to determine whether membrane defects are widespread. An elevated level of creatinine phosphokinase (CPK), which is released from dying muscle cells, is usually a significant indicator of muscular dystrophy and is useful for identifying carriers. If dystrophy is suspected, an electromyographic study determines which muscles are diseased. A muscle biopsy confirms the presence of the disease by demonstrating muscle fibers that are in disarray and contain fatty tissue.[11–13]

TREATMENT

Currently, no effective treatment exists to correct the underlying disorder or to arrest the progression of any of the muscular dystrophies. Steroid treatments were once thought to be helpful, but research has not substantiated any benefits. The primary goal of treatment is to keep the person active and involved as long as possible. Respiratory infections and respiratory failure are controlled through antimicrobial treatment, ventilatory therapy, deep breathing exercises, humidification, and postural drainage. Diuretics are generally prescribed for the cardiac problems. Obesity caused by food intake in excess of the energy demand further compromises these conditions, thus necessitating careful nutritional counseling.

Muscle degeneration and contractures are treated with a variety of methods. Physical therapy is instituted with three goals in mind:

1. to improve muscle strength
2. to prevent and correct contractures
3. to increase the efficiency of functional activities of daily living[3]

Treatment involves muscle stretching, exercise, and the use of adaptive aids. Physical therapists and orthopedists become involved when splints, braces, or surgery are needed. Treatment strategies have also been developed for the specific types of muscular dystrophy. For example, a series of lip, tongue, and palatal exercises have been developed for persons with fascioscapulohumeral dystrophy.[3] Speech therapy may also be recommended for individuals with fascioscapulohumeral dystrophy.

Emotional support of the patient with a terminal illness is extremely important. Psychologists, school counselors, clergymen, family members, and peers all play a vital role in maintaining the person's self-esteem and orientation to reality, particularly when the person becomes debilitated and homebound. Each person must deal with such problems as delayed puberty, depression, dependency, pain, deformity, treatment regimens, financial stress, parental anxiety, and parental guilt.

Genetic counseling is also an important aspect of treatment for the entire family, especially in families in which Duchenne's muscular dystrophy has been confirmed. In spite of the high mutation rate of the gene, mothers and their daughters should be tested to determine if they are carriers, so they can make decisions regarding future pregnancies.

ORAL MANIFESTATIONS

Most studies on the dental implications of muscular dystrophy have focused on the presence of muscular deterioration in the orofacial complex and its resultant effects. Weakness in the masticatory muscles and a decreased maximum biting force have been documented.[14,15] These findings support clinical reports of a higher incidence of mouth breathing, open bite, and overexpansion of the maxilla.[7,16–20] In fascioscapulohumeral muscular dystrophy, the lips appear thickened due to the pseudohypertrophy of the orbicularis oris.[21] Other dental conditions, such as poor oral hygiene, gingivitis, and dental caries, have not been systematically studied but are presumed to increase in incidence as the patient becomes more debilitated and dependent on others for care.

DENTAL MANAGEMENT

The dental implications and home care strategies for persons with muscular dystrophy vary with the type and stage of the disorder. Persons experiencing the Beiker form or a mild form of limb-girdle dystrophy may not require any modifications in treatment, while treatment may be contraindicated in some debilitated patients with Duchenne's form who have severe respiratory and cardiac complications. The basic considerations in dental management involve: (1) ensuring adequate body, head, and jaw stability during dental treatment and home care procedures; (2) preventing further compromises in mental and physical health status as a result of dental conditions or during dental treatment; and (3) assuring that the person's dental health status is meeting his or her functional, esthetic, and personal needs.

Stability and Safety in the Dental Office

Patients with early or advanced involvement of the trunk and neck muscles may slump or exhibit tenuous balance when in the dental chair. Securing the patient with chair positioning, seatbelts, or pillows may alleviate anxiety and facilitate stabilization. Head and jaw support can be achieved by physically cradling the head and using mouth props. The same method should be used by the parent during home care procedures. A patient who can brush unaided may have to stabilize his or her head against a chair or prop elbows or arms during brushing to maintain motor control and minimize fatigue. Long- or large-handled toothbrushes are sometimes easier to manipulate if range of motion or muscle strength is impaired. Patients should be encouraged and expected to participate in maintaining their oral health for as long as physically possible.

Maintenance of stability applies not only to dental procedures but to ensuring the patient's safety in the waiting room, restroom, or during wheelchair transfers. Safety considerations for wheelchair transfers are discussed in Chapter 6. If the patient becomes bedridden and is not easily transported outside the home, a referral should be made to dental professionals who are experienced at delivering dental care to homebound patients. Such arrangements can often be made through the local dental society, dental school, or the National Foundation of Dentistry for the Handicapped. If it becomes evident that a patient will soon be moving from a wheelchair to bed or if treatment is performed in the home, encourage the patient or caretaker to rinse and brush the patient's mouth after meals. Caretakers should be made aware that they may have to assist with oral hygiene needs, but only when the individual can no longer care for his or her own needs. If the patient must be fed, the caretaker should check between the gingiva and cheek for trapped food before and after brushing.

PREVENTIVE MEASURES

In addition to ensuring patients' physical safety, every effort should be made to safeguard their general health status. Long waits in drafty or air conditioned reception rooms or operatories may cause a patient to become chilled, creating increased weakness and stiffness. A patient's inability to close the eyelids tightly due to muscle weakness can be dangerous because of splattering prophy paste, amalgam, water, or other debris. Safety glasses should be provided for such patients. Airway protection is important for patients with impaired cough or gag reflexes to prevent aspiration, which could lead to airway obstruction or pneumonia. Using short, miniscule bursts of water with good suctioning technique will prevent choking. The use of rubber dams may provoke anxiety in patients who feel that their breathing is compromised. Some patients may also prefer a more upright chair position because of respiratory and cardiac problems. Patients who have chronic respiratory congestion may have to interrupt procedures briefly during the appointment to dislodge and expectorate accumulated mucus. The use of foamy toothpaste or fluoride gel for oral hygiene care may also be contraindicated if the person experiences severe respiratory problems.

Dietary evaluation is important when determining preventive strategies and choosing appropriate restorative alternatives. Prostheses, in many cases, may not be practical because of a patient's muscle weakness, impaired chewing strength, and dietary requirements. Patients who consume highly cariogenic foods may require greater topical fluoride supplementation, more frequent brushing and water rinses, and counseling to determine whether other foods could be substituted to decrease the cariogenicity. Many debilitated patients may be eating soft carbohydrate foods that are retained around the teeth and mucosa. Some patients may be on a weight reduction diet that is conducive to dental health and merely need reinforcement for these dietary habits.

TREATMENT PLANNING

Treatment planning is often difficult due to the uncertain prognosis. Functional rather than ideal restorative decisions may be the outcome of choice, but the quality of the treatment should not be compromised. Consultation and joint planning with the physician, patient, and caretaker should form the basis for care. In some cases, esthetics may be important enough for the patient's self-esteem to request extensive restorative treatment. In other cases, maintenance therapy to prevent oral infection is the treatment of choice. The medical status of the patient often contraindicates the use of general anesthesia, so that debilitated patients may also need a maintenance program that stresses optimal oral hygiene to eliminate focal areas of possible infection.

Persons with advanced stages of muscular dystrophy may have speech articulation problems that impair their intelligibility, or they may speak in short slow phrases to decrease fatigue. Effective communication, therefore, can be a frustrating, tedious process that sometimes causes withdrawal or anger on the part of the patient. Dental professionals need to show patience and empathy, letting the patient know that they are listening yet may not be able to understand what is being said. Written messages or nonverbal cues can facilitate communication during dental treatment procedures. Whenever possible, the patient has to play an active role in communicating his or her dental concerns and needs and in making decisions about how these needs will be met.

PATIENT SCENARIOS

Patient 1

Description

John is ten years old and has Duchenne's muscular dystrophy. He is currently ambulatory and attends a regular school. His physician reports that he will be confined to a wheelchair within two years and will require some assistance with self-care activities. John has not experienced many dental problems, but his oral hygiene is becoming progressively worse.

Anticipated Needs

—prophylaxis
—radiographs
—home care instructions
—long range planning

Awareness Strategies

1. What instructions does John need about his home care?
2. How can you help John make the transition to an altered lifestyle?
3. What steps will you take to help John preserve his self-esteem?
4. What guidelines can you help John establish regarding diet?

Patient 2

Description

Michael is 21 years old and is in the advanced stage of Duchenne's muscular dystrophy. He is now bedridden and experiences moderate respiratory and cardiac complications. He cannot chew food well, has no independent self-care skills, yet is still intellectually alert and social. He lives with his elderly mother, who is assisted by a visiting nurse twice a day.

Anticipated Needs

—oral hygiene instructions
—maintenance program
—psychological support
—dietary consultation
—dental referral

Awareness Strategies

1. What program can you plan with the visiting nurse?
2. What can you discuss with the mother regarding diet?
3. What support can you give Michael about his oral health?
4. How will you follow up on Michael's progress?

REFERENCES

1. Smith, M.: To be a man. Companions. Denver, Atlantis Community, 1975.
2. Bleck, E.: Muscular dystrophy, Duchenne type. *In* Physically Handicapped Children: A Medical Atlas for Teachers. Edited by E. Bleck and D. Nagel. New York, Grune & Stratton, 1975.
3. Siegel, I.M.: The Clinical Management of Muscle Disease: A Practical Manual of Diagnosis and Treatment. Philadelphia, J.B. Lippincott, 1977.
4. Adams, R.: Nature and site of lesions in human progressive muscular dystro-

phy. *In* Pathogenesis of Human Muscular Dystrophies. Edited by L. Rowland. Amsterdam, Excerpta Medica, 1977.
5. Adams, A., Daniel, A., McCubbin, J., and Rullman, L.: Games, Sports and Exercises for the Physically Handicapped. ed. 2. Philadelphia, Lea & Febiger, 1982.
6. Conlon, T.: A reappraisal of the proportion of caries and mutation rate in Duchenne muscular dystrophy. *In* Muscle, Nerve and Brain Degeneration. Edited by A. Kidman and J. Tomkins. Amsterdam, Excerpta Medica, 1979.
7. Nowak, A.: Dentistry for the Handicapped Patient. St. Louis, C.V. Mosby, 1976.
8. Dubowitz, V.: Muscle pathology in genetic muscle disorders: some problems in clinico-pathological correlation. *In* Muscle, Nerve and Brain Degeneration. Edited by A. Kidman and J. Tomkins. Amsterdam, Excerpta Medica, 1979.
9. Walton, J.: Progressive muscular dystrophy: structural alternatives in various stages and in carriers of Duchenne dystrophy. *In* International Academy of Pathology Monograph: The Striated Muscle. Edited by C. Pearsen and F. Mostafi. Baltimore, Williams & Wilkins, 1973.
10. Hughes, J.: Synopsis of Pediatrics. St. Louis, C.V. Mosby, 1975.
11. Plishker, C., and Appel, S.: An overview of erythrocyte abnormalities in muscle diseases. *In* Current Topics in Nerve and Muscle Research. Edited by A. Aguayo and O. Karpati. Amsterdam, Excerpta Medica, 1979.
12. Sibert, J., Harper, P., and Thompson, R.: Carrier detection in Duchenne muscular dystrophy: evidence from the study of obligatory carriers and mothers of isolated cases. *In* The Biochemistry of Myasthenia Gravis and Muscular Dystrophy. Edited by C.G. Lunt and R.M. Marchbanks. New York, Academic Press, 1978.
13. Badshaw, M.L.: Children with Handicaps: A Medical Primer. Baltimore, Paul Brooks Publishing Co., 1981.
14. Hamada, T., Kawazoe, Y., and Yamada, S.: Maximum biting forces in patients with progressive muscular dystrophy. J. Dent. Handicapped, *3*:20–22, 1977.
15. Hamada, T., Kobayashi, M., and Kawazoe, Y.: Electromyographic activity of masticatory muscles in patients with progressive muscular dystrophy (Duchenne type): relation between integrated electromyographic activity and biting force. Special Care in Dentistry, *1*(1):37–38, 1981.
16. Brown, J.C., and Losch, P.K.: Dental occlusion in patients with muscular dystrophy. Am. J. Orthodont. *25*:1040–1046, 1939.
17. White, R., and Saekler, A.: Effects of progressive muscular dystrophy on occlusion. JADA, *49*:4–49, October, 1954.
18. Ardran, G.M., Hamilton, A., and Kemp, F.H.: Enlargement of the tongue and changes in the jaws with muscular dystrophy. Clin. Radiol., *24*:359–364, 1973.
19. Cohen, M.M., Sr.: Congenital, genetic, and endocrinologic influences on dental occlusion. Dent. Clin. North Am., *19*(3):499–514, 1975.
20. Kerborg, S., Jense, B., Moller, G., and Bjork, A.: Craniofacial growth in a case of congenital muscular dystrophy: a roentgencephalometric and electromyographic investigation. Am. J. Orthodont., *74*:207–15, 1978.
21. Nowak, A.J. (ed.): The Patient with a Handicap. Iowa City: University of Iowa, 1982. (Unpublished manual.)

Chapter 9

EPILEPSY

The term "epileptic" conjures up an image of a person experiencing fainting spells or lying on the floor having convulsions or "fits." The term epilepsy is derived from a Latin word meaning "falling sickness."[1] Epilepsy has been misconceived through the centuries to be a form of insanity, caused by such things as demonic possession, radioactive fallout, and exotic foods.[2] Persons with epilepsy and their families, in conjunction with the Epilepsy Foundation of America, have been working for years to inform the general public, employers, and insurance companies of the facts about epilepsy. Unfortunately, the public information campaigns have been only moderately successful in changing the stigmata and discriminatory laws associated with epilepsy. As dental professionals, we need to know the facts about this condition so we can provide appropriate, knowledgeable, and normalized dental care to people who suffer from epilepsy.

DEFINITION

The terms *seizure*, *epilepsy*, *convulsion*, and *fit* are often used interchangeably. Each term, however, has a different meaning and describes specific characteristics or conditions, as noted in Table 9–1. Epilepsy is not a disease; rather it is symptomatic of brain dysfunction and is characterized by discrete, recurring behavioral manifestations, which include disturbances of balance, sensation, behavior, perception, or consciousness.[3]

INCIDENCE AND ETIOLOGY

Accumulation of data on the incidence of epilepsy is difficult due to inadequate reporting procedures and under-reporting because of the resulting stigma. Recent studies suggest a prevalence between 2 and 22 per 1,000 population. Wide prevalence rates can be ex-

TABLE 9–1. Definition of Terms.

Seizure:	An episode of cerebral dysfunction produced by abnormal, excessive neuronal discharge; not necessarily a recurring condition
Epilepsy:	A disorder of the central nervous system characterized by repeatedly occurring seizures that result from a storm of uncontrolled electrical discharges in the brain[2]
Convulsion:	Describes a broad range of behavioral manifestations including seizure activity
Fit:	Outmoded synonym for convulsion or seizure[6]

plained by differences in definitions and methodologic procedures employed by researchers. The figures cited by the Epilepsy Foundation of America include all forms of epilepsy and thus are higher than those identified in most texts.[2]

Epilepsy occurs at any age; however, the majority (77 to 90%) of individuals who have epilepsy experience their first seizure before age 20. The onset of epilepsy is highest between birth and four years and during puberty. Several studies confirm that epileptics have a shorter life span than the general population. Higher death rates, especially between the ages of 20 to 55, are attributed to suicide, brain tumors, and accidents.

The causes of seizure activity are numerous and can be described as prenatal, perinatal, postnatal, and unknown.

Prenatal factors include infectious diseases in the mother, fetal

TABLE 9–2. Causal Factors Associated with Epilepsy

Conception to First Two Years	Preschool Through High School	Young Adult Through Old Age
Abdominal trauma	Head injury	Head injury
Premature labor	Whooping cough	Brain tumor
German measles	High fever	Vascular sclerosis
Undetected infections	Lead encephalopathy	Late evidence of birth injury
Difficult birth	Allergy	Other
Congenital defects	Infectious diseases	
Inherited metabolic errors	Brain tumor	
Rh incompatibility	Late evidence of birth injury	
Infectious process (viral encephalitis)	Other	
High fever		
Postnatal trauma (head injury)		
Allergy		
Whooping cough		
Lead encephalopathy		
Other		

growth abnormalities, prematurity, hormonal imbalances or Rh incompatibility between mother and fetus, chromosomal disorders, defects due to the use of drugs or exposure of the mother to radiation, and genetic influences. The actual role that heredity plays in the acquisition of epilepsy is not known. Researchers agree that conditions such as hypocalcemia and endocrine disorders that lead to seizure disorders are inherited, but epilepsy is not inherited. There is an indication of familial tendency.

Perinatal causes include a multitude of potential problems that arise as the fetus begins the birth process, including poor fetal position, anoxia, and the use of forceps.

Postnatal causes include brain trauma due to injury, tumors, prolonged high fever, parasitic infections, and the use of toxic agents, including drugs. Toxic agents cause brain damage by blocking the flow of oxygen for an extended period of time.

No known cause has been determined for approximately 26 to 47% of diagnosed epileptics.[2] Table 9–2 summarizes the numerous causes.

CLASSIFICATION AND SYMPTOMS

Epilepsy can be classified according to (1) site of seizure origin in the brain, (2) etiology, or (3) type of seizure activity. This chapter focuses on the type of seizure activity observed in the forms of epilepsy. These include grand mal, petit mal, psychomotor, and focal or Jacksonian seizures.

Grand Mal Seizures

Grand mal seizures, sometimes referred to as major motor seizures, are the most frequently observed, most clinically defined form of epilepsy, and often the most frightening to observers. These seizures occur at any age and may be preceded by some abnormal sensory activity called an aura, which can include an unusual smell, peculiar sound, feeling of nausea, fear, or tingling sensation. Not all individuals have an aura before a grand mal seizure. People who experience auras may not have one before each seizure.

During the onset of a grand mal seizure, a person suddenly stops all activity, loses consciousness, and falls with boardlike rigidity if standing or sitting. As the individual's muscles contract at the beginning of the seizure, air is forced from the lungs. The outrush of air through the vocal cords may produce the strange noise that is described as the epileptic cry. After losing consciousness, repetitive tonic muscular rigidity begins, followed by clonic relaxation. During the course of the seizure, the eyes may roll back, revealing only the sclera, and breathing may become labored, causing a

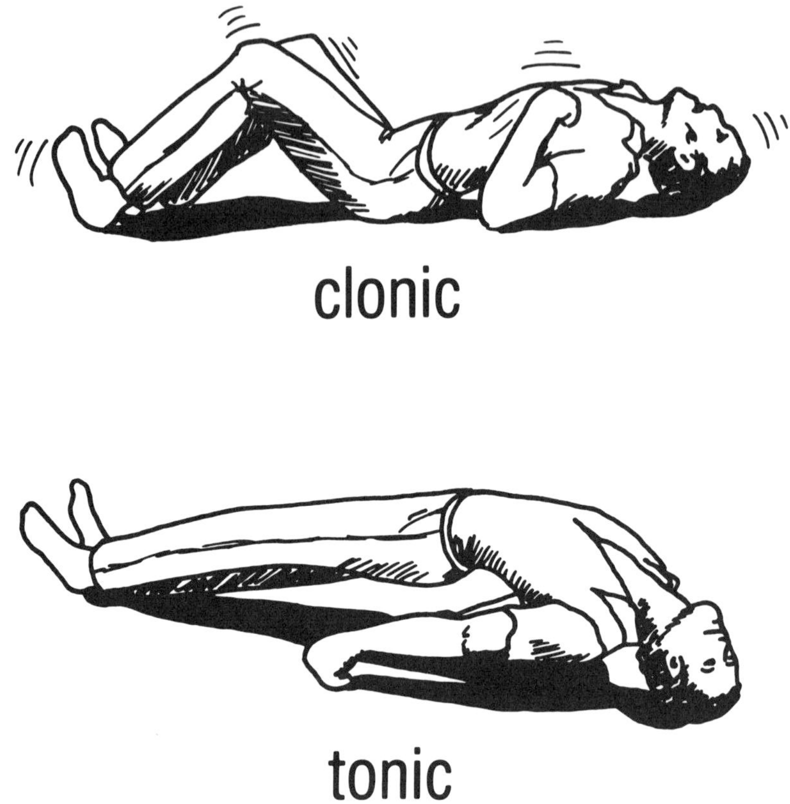

Fig. 9–1. Tonic-clonic action of grand mal epilepsy.

bluish tint to the face, fingernails, or lips. The individual may sweat profusely, drool, and become incontinent, soiling the clothing. The loss of consciousness and repetitive tonic-clonic action of the muscles typically lasts one to three minutes (Fig. 9–1).

Following the seizure, the individual regains consciousness and may be in a confused, frightened state. If the seizure is prolonged (two to four minutes), the individual may experience headaches, nausea, vomiting, muscle soreness, speech impairment, and mental confusion. Some may want to sleep after the seizure. Sleep will last for a few minutes to several hours. After the seizure and a period of rest, the person can carry on normal activities.

The frequency of grand mal seizures varies among individuals. Some people experience an occasional seizure (one per year), while others have several a day. Prolonged seizure activity can produce permanent neurologic damage.[1,3] "Status epilepticus" refers to a grand mal seizure or a series of seizures that last longer than five minutes; it constitutes a medical emergency.

Petit Mal Seizures

Petit mal seizures occur most frequently in children between the ages of 2 to 14. Petit mal seizures usually involve five- to ten-second episodes described as staring, day-dreaming, or unconsciousness without posture loss. Petit mal seizures may last as short as a second, with immediate resumption of the activity the person was engaged in prior to the seizure. The frequency of petit mal seizures varies but may range from 1 to 100 daily. Fortunately, few people experience this many.[1,3] A condition of continuous petit mal seizures, known as petit mal status, occurs but rarely. This condition causes complex, purposeless, stereotypic behavior that is not related to the tasks at hand. Typically, petit mal status lasts only a few minutes; however, the duration may be longer. Between the ages of 10 and 13, about 50% of individuals with petit mal develop grand mal epilepsy. Some develop other forms of epilepsy, while a few cease seizure activity. Isolated petit mal seizures are infrequently observed in persons after the age of 30.[4]

Akinetic attack and myoclonic forms of epilepsy are often included with petit mal epilepsy because of the similarity in electroencephalographic (EEG) patterns. The akinetic form is associated with sudden drop attacks, in which the person loses muscle tone and falls, usually hitting the head. Typically, the person gets up immediately and resumes activities. The myoclonic form involves brief contractions of a portion of a muscle or group of muscles.[5]

Psychomotor Seizures

Psychomotor seizures usually begin in the temporal lobe and typically are manifested by repetitive, stereotypic movements, such as pulling at clothes, lip smacking, chewing, or repeated swallowing. Some people with this type of epilepsy may show aggressive behavior that escalates upon restraint. Most psychomotor seizures, however, are confined to stereotypic activities of which the person has no memory afterwards. Usually the seizure activity lasts one to two minutes and is followed by a confused state. Psychomotor seizures may be preceded by a variety of auras: unpleasant odors, nausea, abdominal pain, peculiar tastes, word phrases, music, or an intense feeling that they have visited a place they have never been (déjà vu). The frequency of psychomotor epilepsy increases with age, occurring most often in adolescence and adulthood. It is the most difficult form of epilepsy to control medically.[5]

Focal or Jacksonian Seizures

A less common type of seizure activity is the focal or Jacksonian seizure. Most often the focal seizure originates in the frontal lobe. The manifestations of the seizure activity depend on the extent and location of the lesions in the frontal lobe. Typically, the motor neuron discharge is localized and affects only certain body parts in specific sequences. For example, one form starts with a clonic jerking movement of a thumb and spreads to the hand, arm, and face. Another form may cause a twitching on one side of the face (usually the corner of the mouth), which is transmitted to the rest of the face. Rarely does a focal seizure induce unconsciousness or result in mental confusion. Seizure activity generally stops shortly after reaching the last muscle group involved. Individuals with focal seizures normally resume their activities after the conclusion of the seizure.[3,4]

Seizure activity does not always fit into the aforementioned classifications. Mixed seizure activity occurs in individuals who exhibit a combination of seizure disorders. Cases have been identified that represent every combination of the four major categories. The most frequent combination is the grand mal and petit mal types of activity. On the other hand, some individuals are placed in an unclassified category because of the confusing nature of their disorder.[4,6]

A seizure disorder should not be confused with a seizure or convulsion that results from drug overdoses, brain tumor, or other problems. All such activity should be medically evaluated.

TREATMENT

Treatment for a seizure disorder is contingent upon a complete physical examination so that metabolic or other disorders can be ruled out. Conditions such as hyperglycemia, mineral imbalances, or a tumor often cause episodic seizures and necessitate differing forms of treatment. Once the presence of a seizure disorder has been confirmed (usually by an EEG study), a program of drug therapy is initiated in about 70% of the cases.[4,5,7] For the majority of individuals, anticonvulsant drug therapy is the only practical long-term treatment.[8] Drug therapy completely controls seizures in about 50% of the cases.[9]

The anticonvulsant drug prescribed varies with the type of epilepsy.[10] The mechanisms of interaction and the prolonged effects of the drugs on the human body are not yet fully understood.[11] Table 9–3 outlines some of the more commonly used anticonvulsants and their potential side effects. Overmedication and drowsiness may hamper effective communication. Drug therapy begins by selecting one drug and administering it in increasing doses until the seizures are controlled or until the blood serum level approaches the toxicity level for that drug. If control cannot be

TABLE 9–3. Common Side Effects of Anticonvulsant Medications

Dilantin:	Gingival overgrowth, drowsiness, skin rash, ataxia, tremors, increased body hair
Phenobarbital:	Drowsiness, skin rash, ataxia
Mysoline:	Drowsiness, dizziness, loss of appetite, nausea and vomiting, blood dyscrasias
Milontin:	Drowsiness, headache, nausea
Celontin:	Drowsiness, ataxia, headache, blood dyscrasias
Tridione:	Hiccoughs, light sensitivity, kidney problems, hair loss, anemia
Tegretol:	Drowsiness, headaches, vision problems, gait disturbances, liver changes, blood dyscrasias
Diamox:	Headaches, loss of appetite and weight, drowsiness, dizziness

Adapted from D.H.E.W. Pub. (HSA) 78-5217, pp. 14 and 15, 1977, and Pediatric Seizure Clinic Pamphlet, University of Michigan, pp. 4 and 5.

achieved with a single drug, a second drug is added after reducing the dose of the primary drug. In about 30% of persons with epilepsy, complete control is never achieved. The goal of treatment then is decreasing the frequency and severity of the seizure activity. Treatment with anticonvulsant drugs usually lasts two to three years after the cessation of seizure activity, at which time the medications are gradually withdrawn.[4,12] Statistics from a recent follow-up study indicate that after three years, one-half of the epileptics experienced complete remission after withdrawal of medication.[13]

Treatment is not limited to anticonvulsant drugs. In severe cases of uncontrollable seizure activity or those in which the focal point of seizure activity can be pinpointed to the temporal lobe, surgery may be indicated. Surgery involves the removal of a single temporal lobe or the destruction of brain tissue with the use of electrodes inserted into the affected area.[3] Dietary regimens involving use of a ketogenic diet and restriction of fluid intake have been successful in some cases, but are generally a controversial treatment modality.

People with epilepsy do have some control over reducing the likelihood of a seizure. They are taught to avoid fatigue, irregular hours, missing medications, or other conditions that lower the threshold of seizure activity. Adults are encouraged to avoid drugs, including alcohol, especially to prevent an adverse drug reaction with their medications. As another preventive measure, some severely involved patients with uncontrolled seizure disorders wear padded helmets to protect them from head trauma. Occasionally these patients wear mouth or chin protectors to prevent trauma to the teeth and gums.

PSYCHOSOCIAL IMPLICATIONS

Problems involved in adjusting to a seizure disorder center around the person's self-concept and the manner in which society helps to shape that self-concept. The stigma associated with having a seizure in public and facing the concerns, questions, and in some cases, the ridicule of onlookers, peers, and friends is sometimes devastating. The denial of a driver's license, military career, or exclusion from hazardous careers are examples of situations that were created to protect epileptics and others. The denial of a driver's license probably has the most far-reaching consequences, causing restriction in career selection, loss of social mobility (especially important to teens), and dependence on others for transportation.[1] Unfortunately, epileptics have been denied employment in occupations for which they were trained simply because potential employers did not understand the condition or were afraid of the reactions or repercussions of the public or insurance companies.[13]

In some cases, parents overprotect epileptic children, not even allowing them to engage in closely supervised group activities, because they feel the situation could be painful or humiliating to the child. Self-images can be enhanced by parents or significant others through helping epileptics accept their disability and its limitations, while identifying and enhancing skills and abilities that are valued and marketable in today's society.

One myth that has contributed to a poor self-image is that persons with epilepsy also are mentally retarded. Yet 80% of the people who develop seizure activity after infancy exhibit average or above average intellectual ability.[3] In most states, epileptics retain their diagnostic label until they have had at least two seizure-free years after they stop taking anticonvulsant medications.

DENTAL MANAGEMENT

The avoidance of potential problems in the dental operatory begins with the patient's health questionnaire.[14] Questions that provide valuable information about a patient's seizure history are outlined in Table 9–4. The information gained from these questions assists the dental team members in treatment planning, appointment scheduling, patient management, and preventive procedures. This information should be updated regularly in case of a change in medication regimen or seizure status. The patient and caretaker can generally provide adequate information. If not, the physician should be consulted. Because of the stigmas attached to epilepsy, many people do not want to reveal that they have a seizure disorder. A sensitive, thorough exploration of the importance of a health

TABLE 9–4. Pertinent Seizure Activity History.

First Seizure:
_____ When occurred
_____ What type
_____ Episodic or part of a seizure disorder

Seizure Disorder (Describe):
_____ Factors that precipitate activity, if any
_____ Presence of aura (visual, auditory, etc.)
_____ Frequency
_____ Duration
_____ Loss of consciousness
_____ Motor behavior
_____ Verbal behaviors
_____ Incontinence
_____ Injuries usually incurred
_____ Resumption of normal activities
_____ How managed by caretaker(s)

Treatment:
_____ How well controlled
_____ Medication(s) being taken (name and dosage)
_____ How often regimen is monitored or changed
_____ Any other forms of treatment
_____ Physician(s) name and phone number

questionnaire and its relationship to dental care often enables self-conscious patients to feel more comfortable when disclosing medical and other information. In particular, the confidentiality of patient records and statements should be stressed. Also it is best if the questionnaire is completed before setting up an appointment. A series of sensitive questions asked prior to treatment could lower the seizure threshold.

The probability of a seizure occurring in the dental office is low; nevertheless, the dental team should be prepared to prevent and manage all types of seizure activity. Some general principles apply to the management of all persons with epilepsy:

1. **Nothing can be done to stop a seizure once it has begun.**
2. **Restraining or attempting to move a patient during a seizure can lead to physical injury to the patient and staff.**
3. **Most seizures are resolved within five minutes.**
4. **Stay calm and maintain a calm manner with the patient at all times. Most seizures are not medical emergencies unless the patient is injured in a fall or the seizure continues for more than five minutes.**
5. **Reassure the epileptic patient that his condition will not compromise the quality of dental care provided or influence your perception of his self worth.**

6. **Careful observation of any seizure activity is necessary for documentation in the patient's dental and medical records.**
7. **If the patient is accompanied by a parent/caretaker, describe any seizure activity that occurs and how it was managed.**

Since the behavioral manifestations of seizure activity vary considerably, management considerations are discussed for each category.

Grand Mal Seizures

Normal treatment procedures should be followed for patients who have a history of grand mal seizures. For example, if a rubber dam is normally used for a procedure, it should be used on the patient with a history of grand mal seizures. However, precautions should be taken to avoid possible aspiration, e.g., tying floss to the clamp. Additional precautions might include the use of a rubber mouth prop to help maintain access and to allow quick removal of dental instruments from the mouth. If the patient has a grand mal seizure in the waiting room or operatory, adhere to the following general rules:

1. Remain calm. There is nothing you can do to stop the seizure. It will last 2 to 4 minutes.
2. Remove objects near the patient that may create injury.
3. If the patient is seated in the dental chair, lower and tilt the chair to achieve a supine position to prevent him or her from falling to the floor.
4. The patient may not experience an aura, in which case you will probably not have time to loosen clothing or prevent the patient from closing his mouth. Forcing objects into the mouth tends to produce more trauma than the actual seizure.
5. Remove instruments or objects from the patient's mouth whenever the seizure allows.
6. If oral secretions are heavy, the use of a plastic saliva ejector or suction tip may be helpful, but should be used with caution.
7. After the seizure, examine the patient for any physical or oral trauma. If soft or hard tissue injury is discovered, provide palliative care. If a tooth is fractured, locate the fragment to prevent possible aspiration.
8. During and after the seizure, do not leave the patient alone. Someone should orient the patient to the surroundings and to the fact that a seizure has occurred. Allow the patient to

rest before dismissing him and reschedule the appointment. If a restorative procedure was in process, the preparation should be temporized.

9. If the patient has experienced incontinence, direct him or her to the restroom.
10. If the patient experiences "status epilepticus" (seizure longer than 5 minutes), summon medical assistance and ask for first aid instructions. The dentist may elect to provide appropriate emergency procedures until medical personnel arrive.

Petit Mal Seizures

This type of seizure activity often is not recognized as such, since it does not involve any major motor activity. The staring or daydreaming spells generally do not interfere with technical dental procedures. Patients, however, may not have heard questions or directions, so that communication is affected. Frequent monitoring of the patient's understanding of what is taking place is important.

Psychomotor Seizures

Manifestations of psychomotor seizures are highly variable, so a detailed history will provide clues to behavioral management in the event of a seizure. The patient may become disorganized, angry, or engage in bizarre hand and arm movements. Keep the patient from injuring himself or others. When the seizure is over, re-orient the patient, and determine whether he or she wishes to continue treatment. Remember to enter a description of the seizure and the actions taken in the patient's record.

Focal Seizures

Patients with focal seizures can tell members of the dental team that a seizure is occurring. All dental procedures should be discontinued until the seizure is finished. This type of seizure should produce only a minimal disruption in the flow of treatment. Treatment can usually proceed after the seizure.

ORAL MANIFESTATIONS AND TREATMENT PLANNING

Two major treatment planning problems are associated with seizure disorders: management of orofacial trauma and gingival overgrowth resulting from the continued administration of phenytoin, an anticonvulsant medication. Orofacial trauma resulting from seizure activity may involve soft tissues, such as the lips, tongue, or buccal mucosa, or hard tissues, such as the facial or jaw bones and teeth. Soft tissue injuries are best managed by thorough cleansing, hemostasis, and wound closure.[15] Antiseptic control of infections may be required in some cases. All instances of soft tissue trauma should be examined clinically or radiographically for underlying damage such as bone fractures.

Dental trauma is observed most often in the anterior teeth. Teeth may be completely avulsed, severely fractured, or merely chipped. Treatment depends on the degree of seizure control, patient cooperation, esthetics, and financial considerations. Fixed prosthetic appliances and sturdy restorative materials are more appropriate for persons with uncontrolled seizure activity that predisposes them to trauma. The choice of restorative technique and material depends upon the potential for fracture, dislodgement, and aspiration. Complicated cases often require an interdisciplinary approach involving such specialists as an oral surgeon, prosthodontist, orthodontist, general dentist, dental hygienist, social worker, and others.

Dental hygienists play an important role by educating the patient to maintain optimal oral care of restorations and prosthetic appliances. Instructions for flossing and the use of bridge cleaners or proxibrushes are important. Communication with and instruction for teachers and caretakers regarding these oral hygiene procedures and first aid procedures for oral trauma are also important. Epileptic patients who routinely wear helmets for head protection should be advised about the use of mouth and jaw protectors attached to the helmets.

Recommendations for management of gingival overgrowth induced by phenytoin are documented in reports by the Academy of Dentistry for the Handicapped and the University of North Carolina.[15,16] The problem of gingival overgrowth has continuing importance in oral health because phenytoin remains the preferred drug for treating grand mal epilepsy. Gingival overgrowth occurs in approximately 25 to 50% of patients who take the drug on a long-term basis (Fig. 9–2). Other anticonvulsant drugs do not seem to cause this gingival condition. A few characteristics of the condition are:

1. No difference exists in prevalence between males and females
2. There is a higher prevalence in younger versus older age groups
3. Degree of tissue overgrowth may be related to dosage and duration of the medication, but the data are inconclusive
4. Overgrowth is generally more marked in the anterior regions and on the buccal surfaces of the teeth
5. Overgrowth does not generally occur in edentulous areas

Studies suggest that plaque and other gingival irritants are nec-

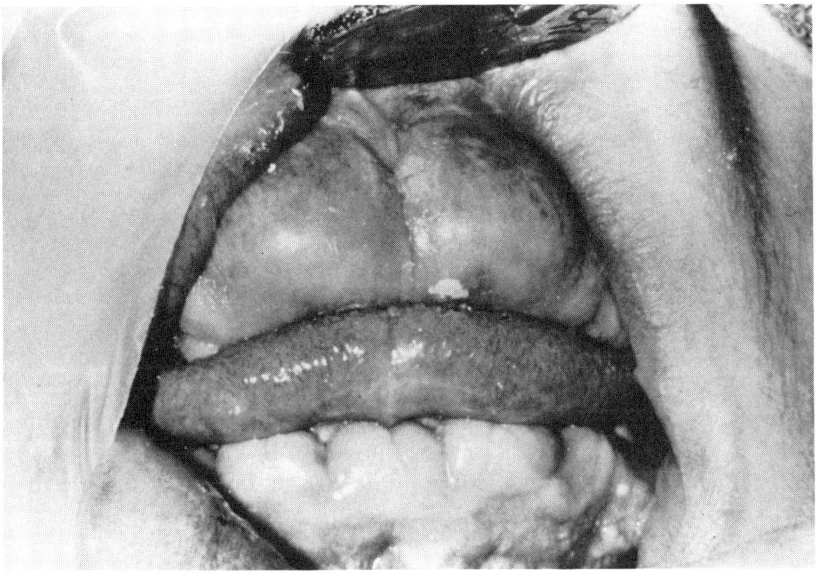

Fig. 9–2. Gingival hyperplasia due to phenytoin.

essary precursors to overgrowth. Any factors that affect the resistance of the gingiva to irritants could also contribute to the overgrowth. Initial studies suggest that a deficiency in metabolism caused by the phenytoin can affect gingival resistance. This situation is often alleviated when physicians and nutritionists prescribe folic acid supplements to prevent the generalized effects of folic acid deficiency.

The tissue overgrowth is characteristically pale, pink, and fibrous, often filling the interdental spaces between the teeth or completely covering the teeth. Malpositioning of teeth, impaired chewing, and compromised esthetics can result. Gingival inflammation is often superimposed on the overgrowth. Effective oral hygiene is difficult due to the configuration of the tissue over the teeth. The tissue can be removed or recontoured through gingival surgery, but will regrow if the phenytoin is continued at the same dosage and the oral hygiene is not optimal. The use of a rubber appliance that is closely adapted to the gingiva and exerts positive pressure reduces the degree of gingival overgrowth.[14] Such a device is usually worn 3 hours each day and all night. Its efficacy also depends on scrupulous oral hygiene through toothbrushing and flossing. Oral irrigating devices have sometimes proved effective in removing trapped food debris from the pockets created by the irregular tissue overgrowth. Fluorides may also be effective in reducing plaque pathogenicity and thereby creating less gingival inflammation.

PREVENTIVE MEASURES

Prevention is the key to the management of patients with epilepsy. As soon as a seizure disorder (particularly grand mal epilepsy) has been diagnosed, parental and patient education should begin. An individualized home program should be developed and a regular in-office recall system established. Frequent updating of pertinent medical information and observation of the patient's emotional status is important for treatment planning and patient counseling. Psychosocial concerns, particularly during adolescence or early adulthood, may interfere with a patient's motivation to adhere to a regular routine or oral hygiene recommendations. Dental health suggestions for alternative oral hygiene strategies and methods for the patient to monitor his own oral health status will help the patient to be less dependent on health professionals. Improvement in oral hygiene can be a positive reinforcer in fostering self-reliance and improving self-image.

PATIENT SCENARIOS

Patient 1

Description

Jim is a 20-year-old who is a new patient at your office. On the health questionnaire he indicates that he has a seizure disorder, but in further questioning refuses to provide you with any more information because "he doesn't feel it is necessary."

Anticipated Needs

—complete medical history
—in-depth interview
—screening and evaluation
—radiographs

Awareness Strategies

1. What is your legal obligation in this instance?
2. How will you establish rapport and communicate with Jim to obtain adequate information?
3. What information should be highlighted in Jim's record?
4. What oral manifestations would give you some clues about Jim's condition?

Patient 2

Description

Melissa is a 10-year-old child with a mixed type of seizure disorder that is resistant to complete control by multiple medications. Her medication regimen is continually changing, and she experiences seizures in an inconsistent pattern.

Anticipated Needs

—parent interview
—complete medical history
—prophylaxis
—treatment planning

Awareness Strategies

1. What discussion should take place among dental team members?
2. What information will you need from the parents?
3. How will you ensure accurate updating of Melissa's records?
4. What will you discuss with Melissa about her condition?

Patient 3

Description

You work in a dental clinic that was constructed in an open bay format to facilitate a team approach and expanded duties of auxiliaries. The patient you are treating suddenly has a grand mal seizure. At the time there are two other auxiliaries, one dentist, and four patients in the clinic.

Anticipated Needs

—emergency plan of action
—protection of patient
—protection of other patients

Awareness Strategies

1. What immediate steps will you take?
2. What are your expectations about the patient during and after the seizure?
3. What precautions will you take for the next visit?
4. What discussion should take place among team members following this episode?

REFERENCES

1. Freeman, S.: The Epileptic in Home, School and Society. Springfield, Ill., Charles C Thomas, 1979.
2. Epilepsy Foundation of America: Medical and Social Management of the Epilepsies. Washington, D.C., 1974.
3. Sutherland, J., and Eadie, M.: The Epilepsies: Modern Diagnosis and Treatment. New York, Churchill Livingstone, 1980.
4. Solomon, G., and Plum, F.: Clinical Management of Seizures. Philadelphia, W.B. Saunders, 1976.
5. Betts, T.: Epilepsy. Brit. Dent. J., *143*:278, 1977.
6. Berg, B.: Convulsive disorders. *In* Physically Handicapped Children: A Medical Atlas for Teachers. Edited by E. Bleck and D. Nagel. New York, Grune & Stratton, 1975.
7. Wyler, A.: Operant control of CNS activity. *In* Epilepsy: A Window to Brain Mechanisms. Edited by J. Lockard and A. Ward, Jr. New York, Raven Press, 1980.
8. Rickens, A.: Drug Treatment of Epilepsy. Chicago, Year Book Medical Publishers, 1976.
9. Adams, R., Daniel, A., McCubbin, J., and Rullman, L.: Games, Sports and Exercises for the Physically Handicapped. ed. 2. Philadelphia, Lea & Febiger, 1982.
10. Chusiel, J.: Correlative Neuroanatomy and Functional Neurology. Los Altos, CA, Lange Medical Publications, 1979.
11. Wilensky, A.: Antiepileptic drugs in the central nervous system. *In* Epilepsy: A Window to Brain Mechanisms. Edited by J. Lockard and A. Ward, Jr. New York, Raven Press, 1980.
12. Lenard, M., and Heslin, L.: The health questionnaire in general dental practice—6. J. Irish Dent. Assoc. *17*(5):168–177, 1971.
13. Epilepsy Foundation of America: Basic Statistics on the Epilepsies. Philadelphia, F.A. Davis, 1975.
14. Goldstein, E.: Convulsive disorders. *In* Dentistry for the Handicapped Patient. Edited by A. Nowak. St. Louis, C.V. Mosby, 1976.
15. U.S. Dept. of H.E.W.: The Dental Implications of Epilepsy. D.H.E.W. Pub. (HSA) 78-5217, 1977.
16. Hassell, T.M., et al.: Summary of an international symposium on phenytoin-induced teratology and gingival pathology. J.A.D.A., 99:652–655, 1979.

Chapter 10

CEREBRAL PALSY

The term *cerebral palsy* was introduced in 1937 to describe a group of conditions caused by one or more brain lesions and characterized by disorders of movement and posture.[1,2] In the past, many dentists and dental teams were reluctant to accept patients with cerebral palsy because of perceived difficulties in communication and controlling patient movement. As a result, many people with cerebral palsy were needlessly hospitalized for dental care. Adjustments are necessary to treat some of these people, yet the procedures are easy to learn and allow the majority of people with cerebral palsy to be treated in private practice or other clinical settings, thus avoiding the expense of hospitalization.

DEFINITION

Cerebral palsy is a static, nonprogressive neuromuscular condition composed of a series of syndromes that result from the same etiology of damage to the brain.[1] The location, extent, and number of brain lesions determine the manifestations. The definition accepted by the United Cerebral Palsy Association states: "Cerebral palsy enhances the clinical picture created by injury to the brain, in which one of the components is motor disturbance. Thus, cerebral palsy may be described as a group of conditions, usually originating in childhood, characterized by paralysis, weakness, uncoordination, or any other aberration of motor function caused by pathology of the motor control centers of the brain"[2] (Fig. 10–1). In addition to motor dysfunction, sensory defects may create learning difficulties and psychological problems. Some cerebral palsied patients also have convulsive and behavioral disorders of organic origin. A primary diagnosis of cerebral palsy, therefore, may be accompanied by secondary diagnoses of mental retardation, minimal brain dysfunction, epilepsy, hearing, vision, and speech disorders,

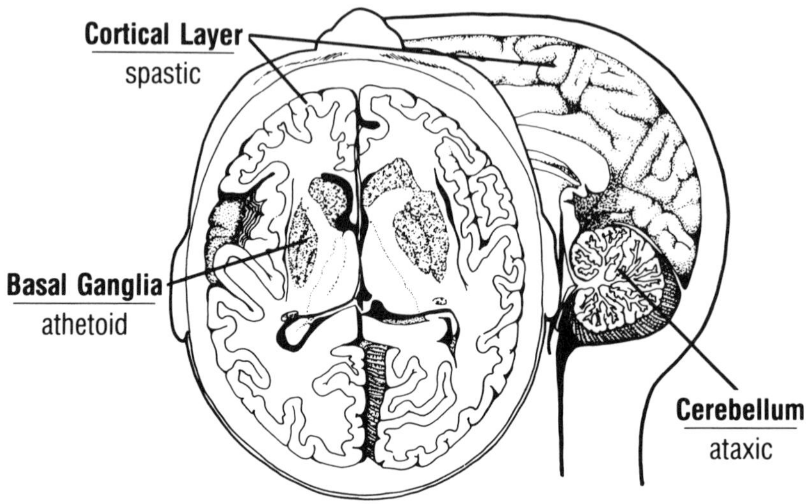

Fig. 10–1. Motor control centers of the brain and the types of cerebral palsy associated with each center.

and several other handicapping conditions (Table 10–1). Of added importance to the dental team are (1) impairments in tasks requiring spatial judgment and orientation, (2) inability to attend to stimuli or overreaction to distracting stimuli, and (3) perseveration, that is, continuation of something (such as repetition of a word) to an exceptional degree.

INCIDENCE

Like many other handicapping conditions, physicians are not required to report cases of cerebral palsy; therefore, accurate incidence rates have to be obtained by comprehensive studies. The currently accepted incidence rate of cerebral palsy in the U.S. is 7 out of every 100,000 people.[3] Cerebral palsy tends to occur more frequently in males than females, although no specific ratio is reported.[4] Marks states that about 10% of people with cerebral palsy are so profoundly involved that they benefit minimally from treat-

TABLE 10–1. Handicapping Conditions Associated With Cerebral Palsy*

Speech/language disorders	60%
Hearing disorders	20%
Visual defects	40%
Mental retardation	40%
Seizures	40%

*Percentages vary with the type of cerebral palsy; these figures are averages from various sources and across types.

TABLE 10–2. Intrauterine and Environmental Insults that Can Lead to Brain Damage

Stage of Life	Potential Cause of Brain Damage
Prenatal	Rh blood incompatibility between mother and child; diabetes in mother; prematurity and anoxia; infectious disease in the mother; uterine bleeding
Perinatal	Onset of labor; anoxia; injury during delivery
Postnatal	Trauma to the head; infections; hemorrhage

ment; another 10% are very mildly involved and need little special attention; the remaining 80% can benefit greatly from specialized training.[5]

ETIOLOGY

Brain damage leading to cerebral palsy can occur as a result of prenatal, perinatal, or postnatal factors. Table 10–2 identifies some intrauterine and environmental insults that can result in brain damage. Some of these factors are of particular concern because of the high incidence of cerebral palsy associated with them. Generally, parents of a cerebral palsied child do not know their child is abnormal until after birth or when the child evidences developmental delays. In only a few instances, such as Rh incompatibility, can precautions be taken to prevent the possibility of brain damage. In short, the causes of cerebral palsy are numerous and methods do not exist to accurately diagnose cerebral palsy until after birth.

DIAGNOSIS AND CLASSIFICATION

Diagnosis is reached by comparing the development of a child to the expected norms for its age and conducting clinical tests to establish irregularities in the developmental sequence. These irregularities may represent gaps in the normal developmental sequence or the replacement of the normal pattern by a deviant pattern, such as spastic muscle activity. The severity of brain damage can be ascertained only through observation of symptoms as the maturation process continues.[4] Other diagnostic tools, such as electroencephalograph (EEG), brain scan, or psychomotor test, may be employed to confirm the occurrence of brain damage.[6]

Individuals with cerebral palsy are classified first on the basis of their motor disorders and secondly according to the limbs involved.[1,2] Six categories are used to classify the motor disorders. Table 10–3 lists the six classifications, identifies the area of the

TABLE 10–3. Description of Cerebral Palsy by Classification, Location of Lesion Within the Brain, Percentage of Individuals Within Each Classification, and Physical Manifestations

Classification	Brain Lesion Location	% Within Category	Physical Manifestations
Spasticity	Cortical layer	50–75	Slightest stimulus causes exaggerated contraction; hyperirritability of muscles; difficulty with head control when the body is in the upright position; depending on severity of the condition, inability to use arms and legs to break falls (protective extension); speech possibly affected; chewing and swallowing possibly so impaired that patient drools
Athetosis	Basal ganglia	15–25	Muscles contract involuntarily; involuntary movements slow, with twisting movements of opposing muscle groups; contorted purposeful movements; difficulty in uprighting and balancing; possible difficulties in speech, chewing and swallowing
Ataxia	Cerebellum	about 10	Muscles respond to stimulus but cannot complete contraction that was started; disturbances in postural balance and coordination; lack of balance sensation; difficulty in grasping
Flaccidity or Hypotonia	Motor area of cortex	<10	Unable to respond to volitional stimulus; unable to stand up; usually cannot hold up head; flaccidity (a form of paralysis)
Rigidity	Cortical layer	<10	Increased initial resistance of muscles that gives way with little force; usually quadriplegic
Mixed	Two or more areas	5–10	Two or more types of cerebral palsy appearing in the same person

brain that is damaged, describes the physical characteristics associated with the classification, and provides an estimate of the percentage of people with cerebral palsy who fall within each clas-

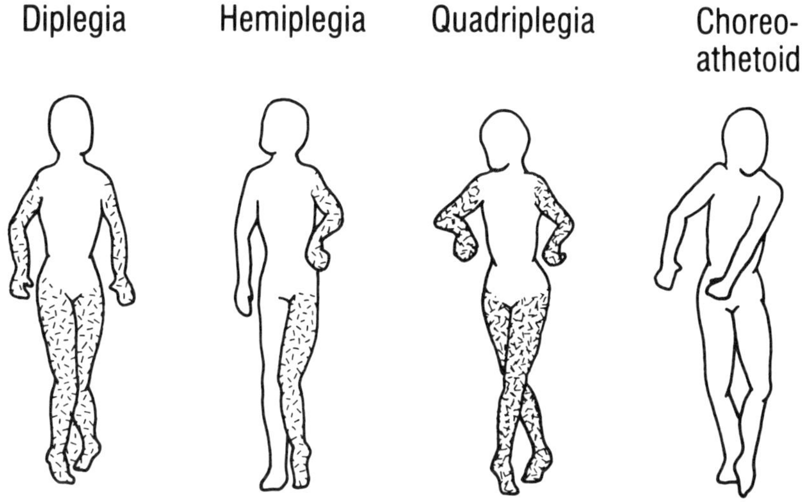

Fig. 10–2. Some types of limb involvement with cerebral palsy.

sification. Limb involvement can be monoplegic (one limb), hemiplegic (both limbs on the same side of the body), paraplegic (lower limbs), diplegic (major involvement of lower limbs and minor involvement of the upper limbs), quadriplegic (all four limbs), or triplegic (three limbs) (Fig. 10–2). Using both classification modalities, a physician's diagnosis may read "spastic quadriplegic cerebral palsy," "athetoid monoplegic cerebral palsy," or any combination of the two classification systems.

TREATMENT

The treatment prescribed depends on the extent of brain damage, age of the patient, symptoms, and the resources of the individual and the family. The goals of treatment include decreasing the severity of the handicap, increasing or improving physical function, providing appropriate education to patient and family, enhancing recreation, and ensuring the best possible emotional life for all involved.[7,8] Treatment can consist of physical therapy, occupational therapy, bracing, orthopedic surgery, speech therapy, medications, and management of any other ancillary handicapping conditions.

The majority of individuals with cerebral palsy can benefit from physical therapy, depending on the type of cerebral palsy and degree of impairment. Most physical therapy programs include daily exercise, usually conducted by the parent at home or by the therapist in a school or outpatient program. Exercise programs are designed to minimize uncontrolled movements while strengthening functional movements and muscles. Adaptive recreation, such as ski programs for the handicapped, also rely heavily on the expertise of physical therapists.

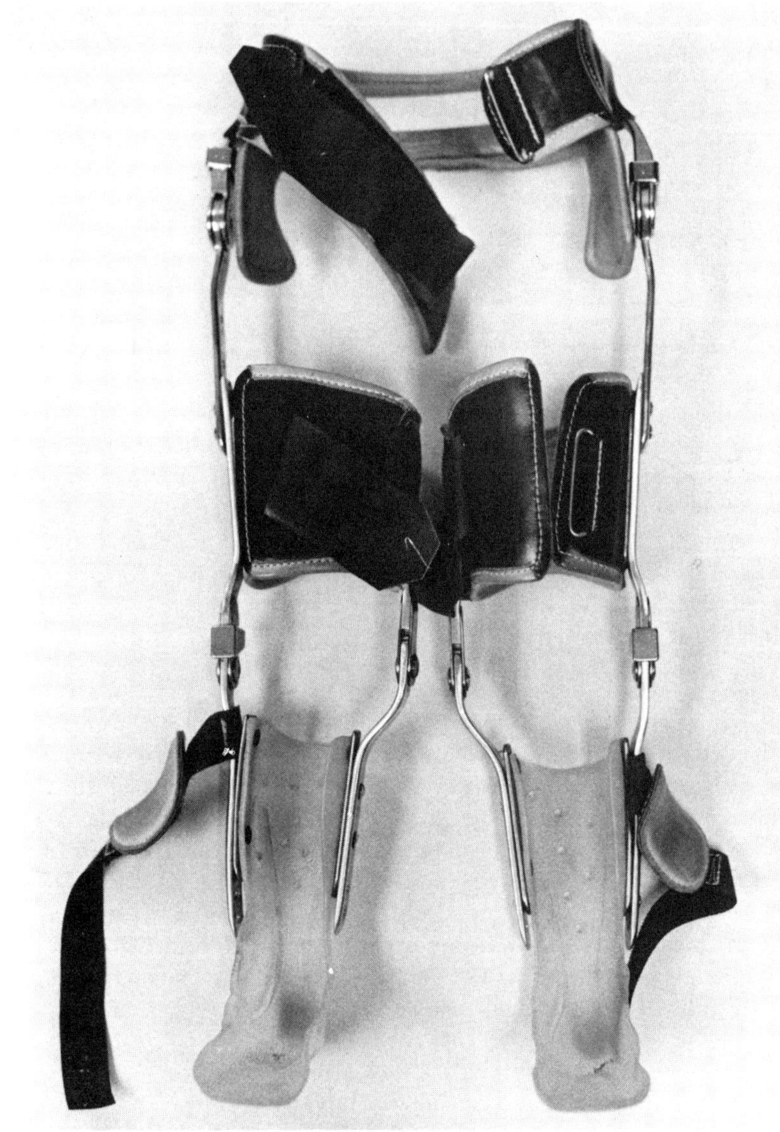

Fig. 10–3. A type of orthopedic brace used to provide support.

Occupational therapy assists individuals in learning new and applying existing skills, particularly those associated with activities of daily living such as eating, dressing, toileting, or on a more advanced level, cooking, laundering, and using transportation. Occupational therapists are becoming more involved in helping these people improve in the areas of sensory-motor integration and visual perception.

Orthopedic braces are sometimes worn to provide support for the body or a limb to prevent further deterioration of the bone structure and loss of muscle function (Fig. 10–3). Braces need to be maintained properly and checked to ensure their proper function and support.

Orthopedic surgery relieves the stretch reflex and muscle contractures by lengthening or weakening muslces. Muscles are lengthened at the tendon and weakened by cutting portions of the incoming nerve.

If speech is affected, a speech therapist works with the individual to improve communication skills. Dummett maintains that the development of speech in cerebral palsied children follows the same sequence as it does with nonhandicapped children; neuromuscular impairment, however, adversely influences the speech musculature. The muscular impairments result in defects in articulation and arrhythmic speech. The development of speech and language can also be affected adversely by perceptual and sensory defects associated with brain damage. As a result, word concept associations develop late.[9] Depending on the severity of the speech and language disorder, treatment ranges from refinement of verbal communication to the establishment of alternative forms of communication, such as hand signing or visual bonding, whereby the person communicates by pointing to a picture in a book or to one of a series of pictures or words on a communication board (Fig. 10–4).

Several medications, such as diazepam (Valium), dextroamphetamine (Dexedrine), chlorpromazine (Thorazine), and methylphenidate (Ritalin), have been used successfully to reduce the adverse muscular effects of cerebral palsy, particularly in spastic and athetoid patients. Barbiturates, on the other hand, have heightened the excitability of some cerebral palsied patients. If epilepsy is present, the person may be taking a combination of medications designed to control the seizure and muscle activity.

The patient may require correction of anatomic structures that interfere with the development of speech. The dental team may be asked to fabricate mouth sticks (see Fig. 6–2). To allow severely

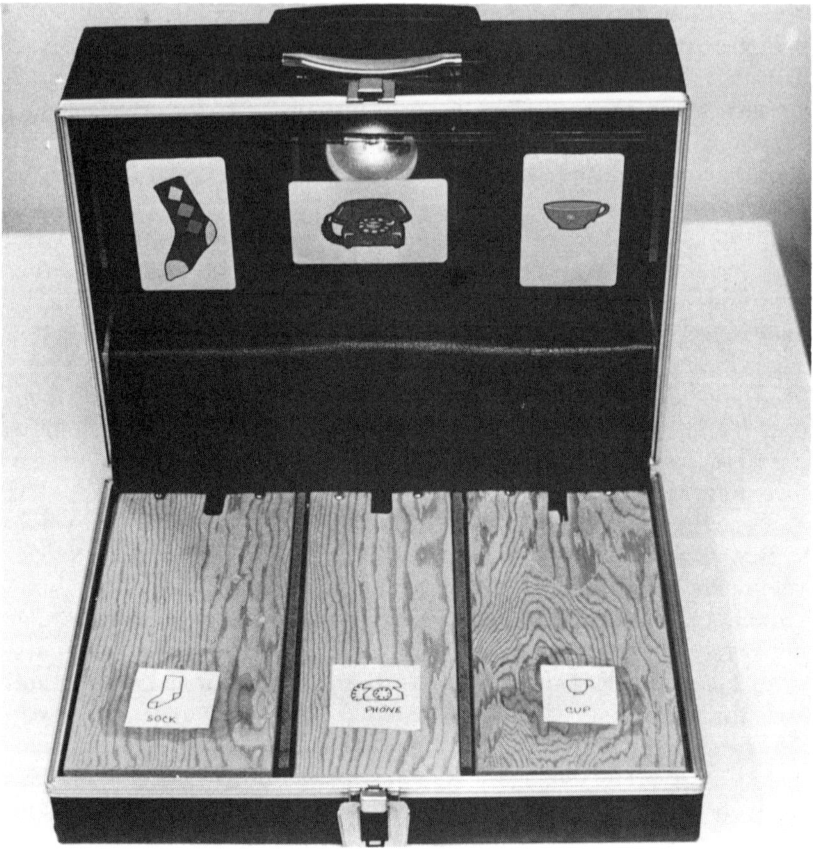

Fig. 10–4. A communication board used by cerebral palsied patients who cannot use language to communicate.

involved individuals to use typewriters, turn pages in books, and accomplish a host of other tasks.[9–11]

PSYCHOSOCIAL IMPLICATIONS

Environment contributes significantly to a child's emotional development. Children with cerebral palsy are constantly reminded of their physical limitations by the environment and by their peers. More often, they are characterized by "what they cannot do" than by what they do well.

Parental overprotectiveness is common and well documented in families with cerebral palsied children. Prior to the development of early stimulation programs, many of these children were kept in rooms devoid of stimulating materials because of fear of injury. Other common parental reactions include guilt, resentment, rejection, denial, depression, confusion, and anxiety.

Self-concept in a cerebral palsied child is molded by all these factors, resulting in a child who sometimes describes him or herself as a nuisance, is embarrassed by his or her condition and by parental overprotectiveness, and is frustrated because of his or her limitations. Occasionally these children become angry, depressed adults who require counseling to maintain a balanced emotional state. The rigors of therapy also influence a person's emotional status, particularly since therapies are often forced, tiring routines.

Because of their compromised physical status, people with cerebral palsy are often assumed to be mentally retarded. In fact, only one-third to one-half of the individuals with cerebral palsy are mentally retarded. Many people with cerebral palsy are highly intelligent people in influential spheres of society. The stereotypic impression of delayed cognitive skills further contributes to the problems these persons encounter in social, educational, and vocational situations.[13]

ORAL MANIFESTATIONS

Patients with cerebral palsy exhibit a higher incidence of bruxism, tooth clenching, dental caries, hypoplastic tooth enamel, periodontal disease, and occlusal problems. Variation among individuals, however, is marked.[10,13,14] The oral manifestations observed in some patients can be related to the severity of brain damage. It has been found that abnormal dental wear caused by bruxism is closely related to a low level of mental development, not to the degree of severity of cerebral palsy.[15] A survey of 119 children with cerebral palsy revealed no relation between the type of cerebral palsy, hypoplastic enamel, or incidence of dental caries, except when Rh incompatibility was responsible for the brain damage.[14] A study of 316 patients with cerebral palsy showed no statistical difference between the spastic, athetoid, and ataxic classifications in terms of caries or periodontal disease.[16]

Numerous studies comparing the caries rate of people with cerebral palsy to control groups have reported varying results. The higher DMF (Decayed, Missing, and Filled) rates generally show a greater percentage of untreated carious lesions and missing teeth due to caries. The higher rate of periodontal disease related primarily to oral hygiene status, which is influenced by the person's level of self-care skills, reliance on others, and the presence of phenytoin-induced gingival overgrowth.[12,13,17,18] Other factors such as food retention due to oral motor dysfunction, bruxism, and increased mouth breathing also appear to be contributory.

These patients also exhibit a higher rate of occlusal problems.

Malocclusion is attributed to abnormal function of the facial, masticatory, and lingual musculature. Like bruxism, the more severe cases of malocclusion reportedly occur with the more severely brain damaged.[19] Tongue thrusting and drooling, caused by abnormal muscle function and impaired swallowing, may accompany the malocclusion.[20,21] In addition, uncoordinated ambulation, frequent falls, protrusive maxillary anterior teeth, and lack of lip protection in some individuals increase the potential for damage to the maxillary central incisors and for subsequent malocclusion.

Hypoplastic enamel characterized by a chalky appearance or irregular surface has been observed in 35 to 60% of cerebral palsied patients and appears to be related to prenatal, neonatal, or postnatal damage to the brain and teeth. These hypoplastic defects in the primary dentition can help determine when the brain damage occurred.

Speech problems do exist for many people with cerebral palsy; however, correction of malocclusion may have little or no effect on the production or articulation of speech. The speech disorders are often linked to the neurologic damage and not the structures used in speech.

DENTAL MANAGEMENT

People with cerebral palsy traditionally have been viewed as uncooperative or difficult to manage. Consequently, few private practitioners were willing to treat these patients in their offices. Recent developments discussed in Chapter 1 have helped to alleviate this problem. Barriers to care still exist, however. Because of previous unsatisfactory experiences with dental professionals, many cerebral palsied persons or their parents are hesitant to return for dental care. Psychosocial concerns such as anxiety, embarrassment, or depression also prevent patients from seeking care. Financial stress caused by medical and other costs is a common barrier. Fraternal groups such as the Grotto Clubs of North America have long recognized this problem and provided financial or dental treatment resources to many patients with cerebral palsy. Transportation is another concern since many patients are confined to wheelchairs or, if ambulatory, may not be able to drive or afford an automobile. Educational and vocational programs, family responsibilities, or other therapies may interfere with appointment scheduling or perception of dental care as a priority.

After potential barriers have been surmounted and a dental appointment is scheduled, certain information should be obtained for planning the first appointment:

1. severity of motor involvement
2. mobility status (ambulatory versus confined to a wheelchair)
3. presence of other disabilities or medical problems and their severity
4. name and phone number of physician
5. identification of who will accompany patient
6. how patient communicates
7. the patient's school or work setting

Risk Factors for Dental Management

Once the patient arrives at the office, the receptionist or other team member can observe the patient in the waiting room and explain customary first appointment procedures. An initial interview with the patient, parent, or caretaker can reveal abnormal muscle and reflex patterns, problems with communication and comprehension, medications being taken, and medical problems.

Abnormal Muscle and Reflex Patterns. Abnormal muscle responses in some cerebral palsied patients are involuntary responses or reflexes often triggered by positioning the patient in the chair or requesting the patient to turn his or her head. The tonic labyrinthine reflex and the asymmetric tonic neck reflex are frequently observed in spasticity and athetosis. The tonic labyrinthine reflex occurs when the head tilts backward. As the neck loses support, the body goes into full extension, the arm reaches out in what appears to be a grabbing motion, then extends and stiffens, as do the legs (Fig. 10–5). This reflex occurs most often when transferring the patient from a wheelchair or placing the dental chair in a supine position. Extension of the back and legs interferes with body support and balance. Extension of the arms and neck interferes with gaining physical and visual access to the oral area.

The asymmetric tonic neck reflex occurs when the head turns to the side or moves away from the midline of the body. As the head turns, the arm and leg on the face side extend and, in some cases, straighten and stiffen. As these limbs extend, the other arm and leg flex (Fig. 10–6). It is important to keep this reflex in mind since most dental treatment is usually performed with the patient's head turned in a variety of positions to facilitate operator accessibility and proper instrumentation.

Lack of coordination rather than involuntary reflexes presents a management problem for the ataxic patient. Ataxic patients react slowly and laboriously, trying to follow positioning and other requests. As they do so, the lack of coordination becomes more pro-

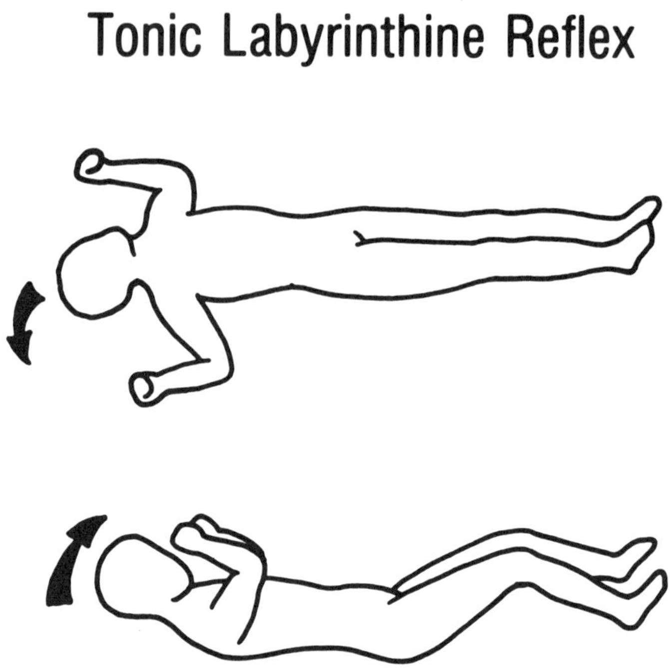

Fig. 10–5. The tonic labyrinthine reflex is triggered when the neck loses support.

nounced and patient stability is difficult to maintain.

The control of muscles associated with movements of the neck, head, mouth, and tongue are of paramount concern to a dental team treating a patient with cerebral palsy. Several devices have been introduced to help the cerebral palsied patient maintain control of muscle activity and reflexes. Harris and Nicholls introduced an automated head stabilizer that attaches to the dental chair. The device reportedly was beneficial, but the expense made it prohibitive for general use.[22] Another item that has been highly publicized but is too costly for a private practice that accommodates a limited number of wheelchair patients is a specially constructed hydraulic base that can receive, raise, and tilt a wheelchair to the appropriate height and angle.[23]

A bean-bag chair placed in the dental chair can help reduce reflex action and provide support during patient positioning.[24] This is accomplished by rearranging the filling material so that the chair molds to the shape of the child, supporting the crucial parts of the body. Although useful for small children, it has limited application for adults.

Much can be done to prevent and control the abnormal movements and reflexes associated with the various forms of cerebral palsy without having to rely on expensive equipment. If a patient is confined to a wheelchair, a decision is necessary regarding patient transfer. Many cerebral palsied patients have joint contractures or other problems that necessiate adaptations to their wheelchairs. Adaptations include adjustable backs, head, chest and leg supports, seat belts, and communication boards. If the patient is well supported and comfortable in the wheelchair and the equipment in the operatory is mobile, certain types of treatment can be performed most easily with the patient in the wheelchair. Patients who require transfer to the dental chair should be consulted regarding the preferred method of transfer. Parents are often more comfortable about transferring the patient themselves than having to explain the procedure to the dental staff. Dental team members should be prepared, however, to transfer the patient or assist if needed.

Once in the chair, the patient can be stabilized with pillows, soft

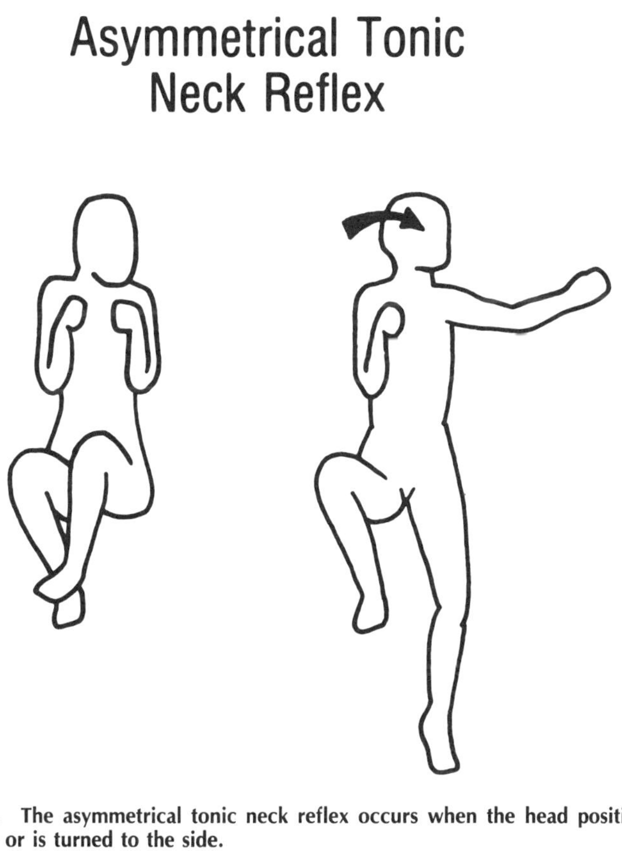

Fig. 10–6. The asymmetrical tonic neck reflex occurs when the head position leaves midline or is turned to the side.

ties, belts, or other methods. Some dental chairs in specialty clinics for handicapped patients are equipped with seat belts. All of these devices should be introduced and explained to the patient and parent as stabilizing devices and supports to facilitate treatment rather than as restraints. Complete stabilization of the head or limbs may be impossible, therefore requiring positioning or other adaptations by the dental team members. Patients with leg or body braces may require adapted chair positioning, or the braces may be removed. Since startle reflexes may also be exaggerated and easily elicited, quick movements outside the patient's line of vision should be avoided.

The asymmetric tonic neck reflex can be controlled by providing treatment from a rear operating position and cradling the patient's head and jaw in the operator's arm and hand. This position alerts the provider to any sudden head movements and enables stabilization of the head in the midline of the body. Treatment that cannot be provided from a rear position may necessitate the assistance of another person for head support. If an asymmetric tonic neck reflex does occur, slowly place the patient's face in midline, help to flex the extended arm and leg, and provide encouragement for attempting the procedure again. The tonic labyrinthine reflex can be avoided by keeping the patient's head supported and flexed, hands folded at the midline of the body, and maintaining the dental chair in a more upright position. If, for some reason, a patient goes into full extension, raise the dental chair, gently massage the patient's shoulders, slowly bring the arms forward, and separate the legs.

The following oral reflexes or patterns may be impaired or abnormal:

1. gag reflex
2. cough
3. bite reflex
4. swallowing

These can be assessed through observation of oral movements and careful insertion of a mouth mirror in different areas of the oral cavity.

A hypoactive (underfunctioning) gag and cough reflex places the cerebral palsied person at risk for aspiration of oral fluids or foreign objects. The use of a rubber dam is suggested whenever possible for operative procedures, and effective suctioning is mandatory for all procedures. Only small bursts of water should be directed from the water syringe. Ultrasonic scaling may not be feasible unless optimal suctioning assistance is available. Hyperactive gag reflexes pose different problems. The introduction of instruments and other dental apparatus into the mouth create strong gag reflexes that can interfere with dental procedures. Flexing the patient's head so that the chin is resting on the chest occasionally reduces the severity of the gag. Topical anesthetic is not generally recommended for the pharyngeal area in light of the other impaired reflexes.

Swallowing patterns often resemble an infantile swallow with pronounced forward thrusting of the tongue. During this process the mandible may be very mobile and unstable, interfering with careful instrumentation and stable fulcruming. The dental team member should provide as much jaw support as possible while adapting to the swallowing pattern. Interference with the individual's swallowing pattern by inserting a mouthprop or exerting excessive force on the mandible may cause great anxiety to the patient by creating a sensation of suffocation or drowning, particularly if the patient breathes through the mouth.

The bite reflex normally appears as an early reflex that facilitates chewing. In many cerebral palsied children, it persists past the normal age and greatly interferes with the feeding process and oral hygiene care. During the dental procedures, the buccal and labial surfaces of the teeth can usually be successfully treated without triggering this reflex. Insertion of instruments from the side rather than the front of the mouth can often prevent its occurrence. Mouthprops are generally useful for coping with this problem, but can trigger the gag reflex or interfere with the swallowing pattern. Procedures that involve the occlusal or lingual surfaces of teeth, therefore, need to be performed as rapidly as possible. Routine sequences for periodontal debridements may have to be altered.

Comprehension and Communication Concerns. Since many cerebral palsied people exhibit sensory deficits, speech and language problems, and mental retardation, comprehension and communication problems frequently occur. Determination of the patient's cognitive level and most effective communication methods prior to initiation of any dental procedures is important. Involving the parent or person accompanying the patient is generally beneficial for assessing these during the first appointment. Their involvement can provide valuable information useful in the management of the patient. Many cerebral palsied patients can communicate by means of language, but their speech is often slow and difficult to understand. Adequate communication may necessitate longer appointments and reduction of noise in the operatory. The number of people trying to communicate with the patient should also be minimized. Suggestions for coping with any visual or hearing deficits are included in the chapters on Visual and Hearing Impairments.

Cerebral palsied individuals generally are able to understand concepts better than they can express them. Their intellectual capacity is often underestimated. Use of specific, clear language does not always necessitate a change in the level of language or in tone of voice. Too often, cerebral palsied adults are spoken to in a childish, sing-song voice because their physical condition and language deficits portray them as helpless, dependent people. Use of audiovisual aids and gestures often facilitates appropriate, effective communication.

Medical and Medication Problems. A comprehensive medical history review and physician's consultation will prevent unnecessary sequelae from any medical problems the patient may exhibit. Since seizure disorders are common, the guidelines for seizure disorders outlined in Chapter 9 should be followed. Persons receiving multiple medications should be carefully monitored if dentally related drugs are used for behavioral management. Some individuals may have hydrocephalus, a condition in which cerebrospinal fluid accumulates in the skull, causing enlargement of the head. This disorder is treated by the insertion of a valvular shunt that drains the fluid to other portions of the body. Such individuals should receive prior to dental treatment prophylactic antibiotics according to the AHA guidelines to prevent bacterial infection of the valve.

PREVENTIVE MEASURES

Certain factors inherent to cerebral palsy place the individual at risk for dental health problems. These factors include:

1. oral motor dysfunction
2. diet
3. gross motor dysfunction
4. suboptimal fluoride intake

Solutions to these problems depend to a large extent on understanding their impact on the patient and the creativity of the dental team members.

Oral Motor Dysfunction

Oral motor dysfunction consists of abnormal oral reflex patterns or abnormal control of the tongue and other oral structures. Inadequate control of oral structures leads to incomplete removal of food from the teeth, mucosa, and palate, promoting bacterial colonization that results in tissue inflammation and enamel decalcification. Simple procedures such as swishing water in the mouth to dislodge food may be impossible for some individuals. Hypotonic lip muscles can also contribute to constant drooling and mouth breathing, leading to increased calculus formation and chronic gingival inflammation with bleeding. Mechanisms for alleviating these problems include:

1. frequent toothbrushing
2. lubrication of the gingival tissue with petroleum jelly
3. fluoride gel applications
4. frequent debridements
5. dislodging food from the palate and mucosa

Occupational, physical, and speech therapists use several techniques to improve oral functioning. Placing one finger gently between the upper lip and the nose and applying pressure will, over a period of time, help the person to maintain mouth closure and swallow more frequently. This is helpful for patients who drool, have their mouths open for extended periods, or swallow infrequently during meals (leaving food in their mouths for long periods of time). The procedure should be employed several times a day as the parent/therapist and child interact and should be performed without telling the child to close or swallow. Digital stimulation of the gingiva also helps to desensitize the child to the touch of a toothbrush. These techniques can be taught to dental auxiliaries who work with severely physically handicapped children, but the procedures must be done consistently and frequently to be beneficial. Dental team members can determine which techniques are being used by the therapists and reinforce them with the child's parents or caretakers. The therapists may be able to provide other valuable suggestions for improving oral function or may actually assist with oral care procedures. Other techniques include the fabrication of mouth props to control bite reflexes or the use of suction devices to remove heavy secretions during toothbrushing.

Diet

Impaired oral function interferes with the development of self-feeding skills and requires the introduction of nutritious foods of different textures. Pureed foods are used with less frequency today for cerebral palsied patients in favor of more fibrous foods that are coarsely grated or chopped. Dietary recommendations for dental health should be given only after a thorough determination of the individual's self-feeding skills, food likes and dislikes, and special diet considerations for medical or metabolic conditions.[25] Consul-

TABLE 10–4. Snack Suggestions for Persons With Severe Cerebral Palsy

Apples (R)	Watermelon
Cantaloupe	Yogurt (regular and frozen)
Orange sections	Cheese (R)
Grated carrots	Seedless grapes
Cucumber	Unsweetened juices
Strawberries (A)	Milk
Peaches	Bananas (R)
Tomatoes (A)	

R = tends to lodge around teeth
A = can be allergenic

tation with the child's nutritionist or physician is recommended. Examples of some appropriate snacks are included in Table 10–4. Snacks for children receiving multiple medications should contain the B vitamins, vitamin D, calcium, and folate because the medications impair the absorption of these nutrients. The usual snack suggestions provided to parents often are not appropriate. Items such as popcorn or nuts are dangerous if aspirated. Prolonged bottle feeding is frequently required for some children with cerebral palsy. The contents of the bottle should be determined and less cariogenic substances substituted if appropriate. Frequent toothbrushing or rinsing of the child's mouth with water is recommended.

Some children may require feeding through a gastrostomy tube, which means that food is never introduced orally. A common misconception is that their teeth do not require brushing. Parents need to be informed that mucus, calculus, and bacteria still accumulate and cause gingival problems, even though dental caries may not develop.

Gross Motor Dysfunction

The approach to home care should be geared to the skill level of the patient. Each patient should be expected to participate to the best of his or her ability. Some require total assistance. Oral hygiene is best maintained by using a manual toothbrush with little or no toothpaste once or twice a day. The manual toothbrush affords the caretaker better control over the area being brushed. The toothpaste can obstruct visual access, impair the individual's swallowing and respiration, and create more of a cleanup job after brushing.[26] If toothpaste is eliminated, other methods of topical fluoride supplementation should be substituted. Disclosing solution is often difficult and messy to use because of frequent drooling. If the parent/caretaker is motivated to use disclosing swabs periodically, a thorough demonstration of their effectiveness is needed. If the parent is resistive, too much prodding can interfere with establishing rapport and decrease the chances for successful parental cooperation. Empathy is much more effective than zealous idealism in this instance.

The hygienist's or assistant's role is somewhat different with the moderately involved cerebral palsied patient. Most of these individuals are able to participate in maintaining their oral health, but require frequent monitoring to determine the effectiveness of their efforts. Brushing techniques for these patients may require modifications to accommodate impaired fine and gross motor skills or retained reflex patterns. Some individuals may benefit from modified toothbrushes (Fig. 10–7) with enlarged handles for improved grip, elongated handles for ease of handling, or angled handles to allow better access. Although there is much written advocating the use of electric toothbrushes, important considerations for these patients must not be overlooked. The electric toothbrush requires a keen sense of perception and control that many patients with uncontrolled movements cannot manage. Indiscriminate use of an electric toothbrush can be dangerous and lead to eye and palate injuries. A productive problem-solving session to try various adaptations is generally the best approach. Flossing is often impossible, but can sometimes be accomplished through the use of a floss holder. Assistance may be needed to thread the holder.

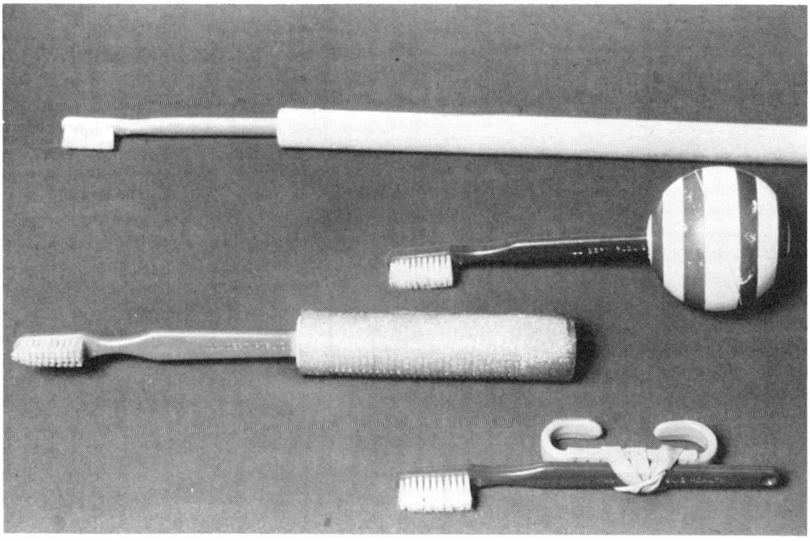

Fig. 10–7. Modifications can be made to toothbrushes to make it easier for cerebral palsied individuals to maintain their own oral hygiene.

For the mildly involved patient, few modifications are required to maintain optimal oral hygiene. The use of disclosing solution is a beneficial educational tool for these patients. The removal of stain in areas where brushing needs refinement will also help in the development of perception and hand-eye coordination. A supply of disclosing tablets or swabs and a chart for recording daily practice of plaque removal should be provided and its use encouraged.

Optimal Fluoride Supplementation

Optimal fluoride supplementation is important because of increased plaque and food retention, an increased susceptibility to dental caries, or other risk factors. Systemic supplementation from water consumption may be limited for individuals who are nonambulatory and depend on others for their water intake. The use of fluoride tablets may be indicated for young children if the volume of water intake is questionable. The most appropriate method for topical administration of fluoride for cerebral palsied individuals is sometimes difficult to determine due to problems with oral motor dysfunction. Mouth rinses are generally not recommended for this reason. Tray applications with gel inevitably trigger a gag reflex. The use of a brush-on gel appears to be the most acceptable method for both home and office applications. Parents should prevent undue ingestion of the gel. Suction should be used in the dental office to prevent ingestion.

The successful management of the patient with cerebral palsy may require more preparation and treatment time than most patients. This time should be anticipated in advance and allocated during scheduling to avoid being rushed. If adequate time is allocated and the team members are prepared for the cerebral palsied patient, the experience can be rewarding and challenging for both the patient and the dental team members.

PATIENT SCENARIOS

Patient 1

Description

Mrs. Benito is a 35-year-old lady who has moderate cerebral palsy, works at Goodwill Industries, and is married to a man with cerebral palsy. She receives regular dental care, but still displays poor oral hygiene and appears to be depressed about her work situation.

Anticipated Needs

— examination and possibly x-rays
— prophylaxis
— oral hygiene instruction

Awareness Strategies

1. What questions might you ask to determine why she appears depressed and how her feelings might be influencing her oral health?
2. What would be your dental health education approach?
3. What treatment modifications might be necessary?

Patient 2

Description

Janie is a 12-year-old child with severe spastic quadriplegia, a seizure disorder, arrested hydrocephalus, and a hearing impairment. She has never had a dental examination because her mother reports that "she bites."

Anticipated Needs

— thorough examination
— full mouth radiographs
— debridement, polish
— fluoride treatment
— restorative care
— oral care instructions

Awareness Strategies

1. How would you communicate with Janie and introduce her to the dental environment?
2. What medical precautions should you consider?
3. What risk factors for dental health problems might she have?
4. What other professionals could assist you in developing a total oral health management plan for Janie? How could each one help?

REFERENCES

1. Bleck, E.: Cerebral palsy. *In* Physically Handicapped Children: A Medical Atlas for Teachers. Edited by E. Bleck and D. Nagel. New York, Grune & Stratton, 1975.
2. Davis, P., et al.: Cerebral palsy. *In* Neurodevelopmental Problems in Early Childhood. Edited by C. Drillien and M. Drummond. Oxford, Blackwell Scientific Publications, 1977.

3. Low, N.: Cerebral palsy. *In* Paediatric Neurology. Edited by F. Rose. Oxford, Blackwell Scientific Publications, 1979.
4. Menkes, J.: Textbook of Child Neurology. ed. 2. Philadelphia, Lea & Febiger, 1980.
5. Marks, N.: Cerebral Palsied and Learning Disabled Children. Springfield, Ill., Charles C Thomas, 1974.
6. Low, N.: Cerebral palsy. *In* Neurology of Infancy and Childhood. Edited by S. Carter and A. Gold. New York, Appleton-Century-Crofts, 1974.
7. Graziani, L., Mason, J., and Cracco, J.: Neurological aspects and early recognition of brain dysfunction in children: diagnostic and prognostic significance of gestational, perinatal and postnatal factors. *In* Brain Dysfunction in Children: Etiology, Diagnosis and Management. Edited by P. Black. New York, Rowen Press, 1981.
8. Adams, R.C., Daniel, A.N., McCubbin, J.A., and Rullman, L.: Games, Sports and Exercises for the Physically Handicapped. ed. 2. Philadelphia, Lea & Febiger, 1975.
9. Dummet, C.: Language and speech pathology in cerebral palsied children. J. Dent. Children, *39*:274–277, 1972.
10. Sorenson, H.: Physically handicapped. *In* Dentistry for the Handicapped Patient. Edited by A. Nowak. St. Louis, C.V. Mosby, 1976.
11. Mysak, E.: Neurospeech Therapy for the Cerebral Palsied. New York, Teachers College Press, 1980.
12. Rosenstein, S.M.: Dentistry in Cerebral Palsy and Related Handicapping Conditions. Springfield, Ill., Charles C Thomas, 1978.
13. Kanar, H.: Cerebral palsy and other gross motor or skeletal problems. *In* Dentistry for the Handicapped Patient. Edited by K. Wessels. Littleton, PSG Publishing Co., 1978.
14. Fever, D.: Dental aspects of cerebral palsy. Dental Student, *49*:43–44, 1970.
15. Lindquist, B., and Herzbel, J.: Bruxism in children with brain damage. Odontologica Scand., *32*:313–319, 1974.
16. Smith, B.: Periodontal involvement and caries incidence in noninstitutionalized cerebral palsied patients. Texas Dental J., *94*:4–6, 1974.
17. Davis, M.: Parotid salivary secretion and composition in cerebral palsy. J. Dent. Res., *58*(8):1808, 1979.
18. Hengen, M.: The role of the dental hygienist in the dental care of the cerebral palsy patient. Dent. Hyg., *54*(10):472–473, 1980.
19. Brown, J., and Schodel, D.: A review of controlled surveys of dental disease in handicapped persons. J. Dent. Child., *43*:17–24, 1976.
20. Moehen, B.: Preventive dentistry for the cerebral palsied—why not? J. Dent. Handicapped, *2*:10, 1976.
21. Rocco, B.: A comparison of temporomandibular joint function in cerebral palsy and non-cerebral palsy children. J. Dent. Guidance Council on the Handicapped, *15*(1):9, 1976.
22. Harris, F., and Nicholls, J.: An automated head stabilizer to facilitate dental care for cerebral palsied patients. J. Hosp. Dent. Pract., *12*(3):92–94, 1978.
23. Posnick, W.R. and Posnick, I.H.: Dental care in the private practice. *In* Dentistry for the Handicapped Patient. Edited by A. Nowak. St. Louis, C.V. Mosby, 1976.
24. Cramer, J., and Wright, S.: The bean bag chair and the pedodontic patient with cerebral palsy. Dent. Hyg., *49*(4):167–168, 1975.
25. Monaco, A., and Beaver, H.: The first dental visit of a cerebral palsied child. J. Mich. State Dent. Assoc., *53*:43–46, 1971.
26. Finnie, N.: Handling the Young Cerebral Palsied Child at Home. New York, E.P. Dutton, 1975.

Chapter 11

MENTAL RETARDATION

We are all aware that members of our immediate family, our friends, and our co-workers have interests, skills, and abilities that differ from our own. Most of us accept and enjoy those differences. It is only when the differences we observe deviate significantly from what we consider normal that we may stare in wonderment, react by withdrawing, or, in a host of other ways, communicate to the person exhibiting the difference that we are uncomfortable. Handicapped individuals often suffer from being considered different and are subject to such reactions from others. The mentally retarded are particularly vulnerable to such "conditional" responses.

The term "mentally retarded" evokes a variety of responses, depending on an individual's exposure to and understanding of mental retardation. Persons with this condition comprise the largest group of handicapped individuals. Consequently, when treating handicapped patients, it is essential that all members of the dental health team understand the concept of mental retardation and are familiar with issues that affect the care and treatment of the mentally retarded.

DEFINITION

The definition accepted by the American Association on Mental Deficiency (AAMD) states that a person is considered mentally retarded if she or he exhibits "significant subaverage general intellectual functioning which originates during the developmental period and is associated with impairment in adaptive behavior."[1] (The developmental period is before 18 years of age.) Stated another way, the mentally retarded person experiences unusual difficulty in learning and is not effective in applying what has been learned to the problems of daily living.

Two types of assessments must be performed before a person is classified as mentally retarded. One assessment focuses on measuring general intelligence; the other, on adaptive behavior ("the effectiveness or degree with which the individual meets the standards of personal independence and social responsibility expected by his age and cultural group"). To determine an individual's general intellectual functioning level, a standardized individual mental measurement test is administered. An intelligence quotient (I.Q.) of 90 to 110 is considered normal or average on standardized intelligence tests. Roughly 50% of the total population falls within this range. People who obtain scores over 110 are considered to have above-average intelligence; those who score below 90 are considered sub-average. The lower the deviation from the normal range, the more serious the mental handicap becomes. The Stanford-Binet and the Wechsler scales are used most commonly to measure I.Q. beyond the preschool age. If people score 68 or below on the Stanford-Binet or 70 or below on the Wechsler scales, their I.Q. places them in the lowest 3% of their peers and their general intelligence is considered significantly below normal.[2]

Maturation, learning, and social adjustment are the three aspects of adaptive behavior that are measured on adaptive behavior scales. These three aspects carry different weights at different ages. Maturation, or the process of normal development, is an important aspect of adaptive behavior in infancy and early childhood. In later childhood and adolescence, more emphasis is placed on the role of learning and social adjustment.[1,3] The performance of an individual on an adaptive behavior scale is reported in terms of a social quotient. If the social quotient falls significantly below the age and cultural group norms, a person would be considered to have retarded adaptive behavior. If an individual has measured deficits in both intellectual and adaptive behavior during the developmental period, she or he is considered mentally retarded.

INCIDENCE

Publications of mental retardation statistics indicate that about 3% of the population of the United States is considered mentally retarded. Recently it has been suggested that this estimate is incorrect. Investigators who examined the standardized tests used to measure I.Q. have found that many of the instruments, with few exceptions, are culturally biased. As a result, members of minority groups may be inappropriately labeled as mentally retarded.[4]

Supporters of the AAMD's multidimensional definition of mental retardation point out that the 3% figure represents only individuals who are expected to fall below the established cutoff points of 68 on the Stanford-Binet and 70 on the Wechsler scales. When the

TABLE 11–1. Approximate Percentage of Mentally Retarded Persons in Each AAMD Classification

AAMD Classification	Approximate % of Mentally Retarded Population
Mild	89
Moderate	6
Severe	3.5
Profound	1.5

criteria of significantly below average *adaptive* behavior are applied, the 3% figure drops to 1%.[5]

Specialists in the field of mental retardation, therefore, disagree about the number of people who should be classified as mentally retarded. If the lower (1%) and upper (3%) estimates are used as guidelines, however, between 2.3 million and 6.7 million Americans are considered mentally retarded.

CLASSIFICATION

The degree of mental retardation varies among those classified as such. The categories of mild, moderate, severe, and profound are used most often to describe the extent of impairment. A varying number of individuals fall into each category. A listing of the AAMD classification systems, with the percentage of individuals in each classification, is presented in Table 11–1.

Proponents of the classification system indicate that appropriate training programs cannot be developed if the skill level of the individual is not determined.[6] Opponents state that labels tend to divide people into groups that are typically thought of as similar, but different from other groups.[7] The effects of classification or labeling can be minimized by developing an individualized educational program that establishes goals that are systematically monitored and revised as needed.[8]

ETIOLOGY

The causes of mental retardation fall into three categories: acquired, inherited, and unknown. Brain damage resulting in mental retardation may be acquired prenatally, postnatally, or any time during the developmental period. During pregnancy, the fetus is susceptible to infections and trauma incurred by the mother. Viral infections that might cause brain damage include rubella (German measles), influenza, cytomegalovirus, and syphilis. Injuries to the fetus may occur as a result of trauma, Rh incompatibility, alcohol

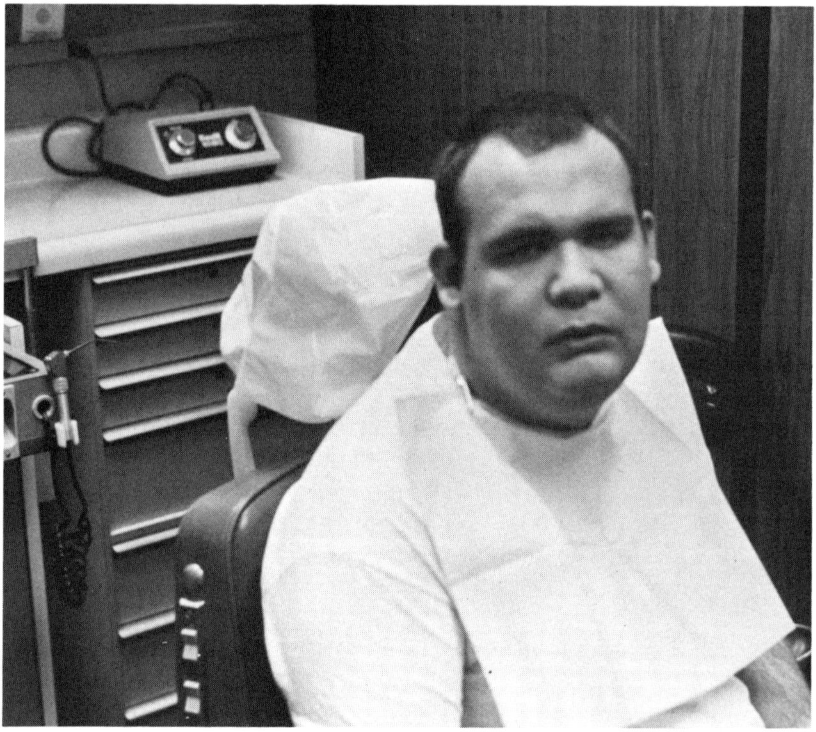

Fig. 11–1. Trauma during the birth process resulted in brain damage for this patient.

consumption, poor nutrition, toxemia, and ingestion of prescribed and nonprescribed drugs.

Trauma during birth may result in sufficient brain damage to cause mental retardation. The most frequently observed forms of perinatal trauma result from difficult deliveries, anoxia, and prematurity (Fig. 11–1).

Postnatal causes of mental retardation include infections that result in meningitis, encephalitis, extremely high fever (105° F and above for extended periods of time), physical injury to the head, and social deprivation (lack of sufficient stimulus to allow a child to learn). Adverse prenatal, perinatal, and postnatal conditions account for approximately 9% of those individuals classified as mentally retarded.

An individual's intellectual potential can be evaluated when inherited metabolic disorders and chromosomal aberrations occur. Phenylketonuria (PKU) is a genetically determined metabolic disorder. Individuals with this disorder are not able to transform phenylalanine (a protein substance) into usable tyrosine. As a result, excess phenylalanine circulates in the bloodstream and causes severe brain damage. Successful prevention of brain damage in such individuals has recently been instituted through dietary management. Chromosome aberration refers to a deviation or variations in the 46 chromosomes normally present in each body cell. For example, the addition of an extra chromosome (no. 21) to each cell results in a condition known as Down's syndrome (Fig. 11–2). Individuals with Down's syndrome may have limited cognitive potential along with distinctive structural abnormalities of the face and limbs. Genetic disorders account for about 13% of individuals classified as mentally retarded.

No specific etiology can be identified for the majority of those classified as mentally retarded (about 75%)[3,9–12] (Fig. 11–3). Unfortunately, not knowing the etiology limits the development of preventive strategies.

PREVENTION AND TREATMENT

Advances in diagnostic, preventive, and therapeutic biomedical techniques over the last 20 years have introduced the concept of

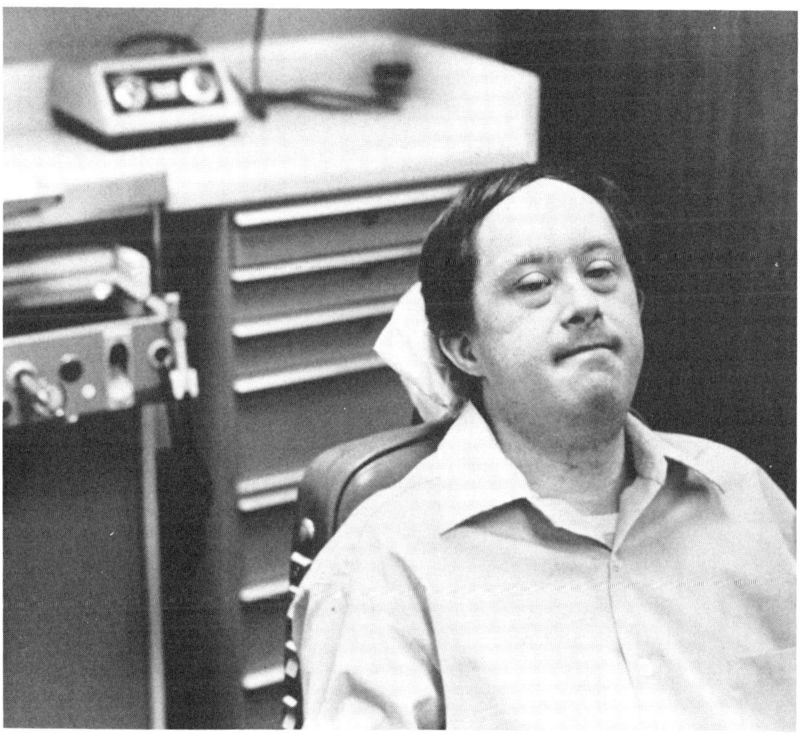

Fig. 11–2. This patient has a chromosome aberration called Down syndrome.

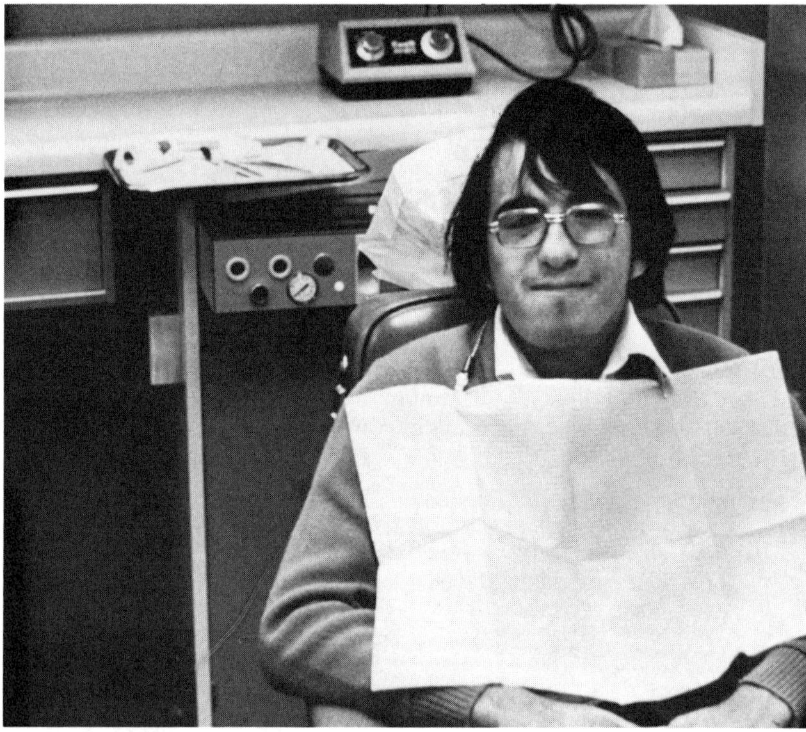

Fig. 11–3. No specific cause can be identified for the majority of individuals classified as mentally retarded, such as this patient.

prevention to the field of mental retardation. Public education programs have been developed to inform expectant mothers about possible adverse effects on the fetus resulting from medications, other drugs (including alcohol), and poor diet. Genetic counseling programs have been established to identify and counsel carriers of genetic disorders that may result in mental retardation or other handicapping conditions. Women who choose to have children but are at risk can undergo amniocentesis after the fourteenth week of pregnancy. This is a process of obtaining fetal cells with a syringe passed through the abdominal wall. The cells can be cultured and examined for genetic disorders. In some instances the fetal growth may be monitored to administer appropriate nutrients or medication that can control chemical imbalances that would otherwise negatively influence the fetus. If the genetic disorder cannot be controlled by such procedures, the parents have the option, in some states, of aborting the fetus or allowing the pregnancy to continue to full term.

If amniocentesis is not available or practical, tests conducted shortly after birth can determine whether certain metabolic disorders such as PKU exist. If such metabolic disorders are detected, the appropriate treatment can sometimes be initiated in an attempt to avoid mental retardation.

The majority of mentally retarded persons are identified after an apparently normal pregnancy and a normal delivery. Education for individuals diagnosed as mentally retarded should begin as soon as possible and should be centered around the assessed intellectual and social needs of the individual. Educational and vocational training are most effective when individualized, monitored, and periodically adjusted to meet the changing needs of the person.[7,8]

IMPLICATIONS FOR DENTAL CARE

Since mentally retarded individuals exhibit such a wide range of needs and abilities, no single approach to the provision of dental care will suffice. Scheduling of appointments, home care suggestions, and treatment plans depend, to a certain extent, on the person's living arrangements, school or work program, participation in supportive services such as speech, physical, or occupational therapy, and any medical, emotional, or other problems that compound the mental impairment.

Depending on the etiology of the mental retardation, the patient may exhibit or report a variety of medical problems. Some patients with Down's syndrome reportedly have an increased incidence of hearing disorders, congenital heart problems, leukemia, and obesity. Seizure disorders are not uncommon in persons with mental retardation. Organ systems such as the kidney or liver may be damaged if the child has multiple birth defects. If a patient has been diagnosed as having a specific type of condition or syndrome that contributes to or caused the mental retardation, a review of the condition or syndrome is useful for determining which medical problems can be anticipated. Multiple medications are commonly taken by some patients who demonstrate behavioral problems in addition to medical problems.

ORAL MANIFESTATIONS

Most dental problems in persons with mental retardation are not inherent to the disability, but are related to extrinsic factors associated with the condition.[13] Although the incidence of dental caries appears to be no higher than that in the general population, the high percentage of untreated carious lesions reported in the literature is primarily a reflection of personal and professional neglect.[14–16] A high incidence of gingival and periodontal disease is reported and is probably related to poor oral hygiene practices and infrequent professional debridements.[12,14,15] Malocclusion tends to occur more frequently in those mentally retarded persons who exhibit craniofacial syndromes or extreme gingival overgrowth from phenytoin.[14] Developmental anomalies of the enamel, such as hypocalcification and hypoplasia, have been noted in some individuals.[17,18] Patients with Down's syndrome may exhibit several dental conditions, including enamel dysplasia, reduced tooth and root size, delayed tooth eruption, early developing and refractory periodontal disease, reduced caries rate, and differences in craniofacial proportions that affect occlusion.[19,20]

DENTAL MANAGEMENT

Initial Contact

Persons with mental retardation may call for a dental appointment themselves or rely on parents, caretakers, or others to arrange dental care for them. Many mildly retarded persons who schedule their own appointments may not inform you of their condition, and members of the dental team may never be aware that these patients have been classified as mentally retarded.

When the person who schedules appointments becomes aware that a potential patient is mentally retarded, the following information should be gathered:

1. age and functioning level of the patient
2. presence of other handicapping conditions and their nature
3. the person's mobility status (e.g., ambulatory vs. need for a wheelchair)
4. previous dental care exposure and possible management problems
5. reason for the appointment
6. responsible party for financial and consent purposes

This information will help the team to prepare for the first appointment. If the patient appears to have a complicated medical history, the medical and dental history forms can be sent home for completion with instructions to bring them to the first appointment. This process enables group home counselors or caseworkers to review charts or records and provide accurate information rather than having the patient arrive at the office with inaccurate or inadequate information. Valuable dental staff time is also saved.

First Appointment

Shortly after arriving for the first appointment, the patient, along with the parent(s), legal guardian, or agency representative, should be admitted to an office or operatory where a member of the dental team obtains or reviews the health history. Of particular note should be information about medications currently being taken, other handicapping conditions, living arrangements, education or employment status, and primary caretaker. This is the time to observe and interact with the patient to determine communication skills, reaction to the dental office environment, and emotional status. If the patient is fearful, withdrawn, or unable to communicate effectively, the person who accompanies the patient should be asked to help provide reassurance and serve as communicator. Individual circumstances, office layout, and professional preference determine whether this person should be present in the dental operatory during the entire appointment.

After the health history has been obtained, the patient should be seated in the dental chair and his or her attention directed to the team member conducting the examination. If other patients or dental staff are present in the same room, they should be acknowledged or introduced so that the patient is not distracted or confused.

The dental team member can enhance communication with the patient through a tell-show-do technique. It is important to review all procedures to be performed during the first appointment and then explain each one separately as it occurs. The patient should be allowed to explore and ask questions about the chair and other equipment. This includes an introduction to the sounds of the equipment and the operation of the air and the water syringe prior to their actual use. The use of the syringe, handpieces, and instruments can be demonstrated first on the dental staff and then on the patient. The patient's understanding of the equipment can be assessed by his or her calmness or agitation. If necessary, a slower pace or redemonstration should be initiated.

During the oral examination, the patient may wish to observe procedures with a hand mirror. Dental charting can be introduced as "counting and feeling the teeth." Oral hygiene assessment and instruction often serve as easy introductory procedures for first appointments. All procedures should be accompanied by positive verbal and physical reinforcement. This means smiling, touching the patient's hand or shoulder, and allowing the patient to touch, hold, or feel certain pieces or instruments. Early assessment of oral hygiene facilitates treatment planning and provides an opportunity to assess the patient's or caretaker's understanding of and motivation for preventive dental procedures.

If the oral examination proceeds well, radiographs may be attempted. Strong consideration should be given to obtaining only those radiographs necessary for diagnosis, using appropriate shielding devices such as lead aprons. A quality radiographic survey is often the most difficult procedure to accomplish, since it requires the patient's utmost cooperation, and the films may cause excessive gagging.[21] If the patient becomes restless or distressed during this process, postpone it and review another procedure in which success was experienced to reinforce the patient's cooperation and conclude the visit on a positive note. Provide the patient with a new toothbrush at the end of the visit.

Second and Subsequent Appointments

The second appointment should begin by reviewing what was accomplished during the first appointment. In most cases, a treatment plan can be presented to the patient or to the parent, guardian, or other responsible person. Before beginning treatment, or in the event that the treatment plan needs to be altered, an informed consent should be obtained.[22] The informed consent gives the dental team permission to perform the procedures identified in the treatment plan. The patient or his legal representative has the right to consent to or refuse all or any part of the treatment.[23]

Periodontal debridement and polishing are the optimal procedures to be performed at the second appointment unless the patient is in pain. These procedures prepare the oral cavity for future procedures by removing local irritants and enhancing tissue health. Oral hygiene should also be checked and home care procedures reinforced at this time.

If the patient does not respond positively to verbal behavioral management techniques and treatment cannot proceed, the use of premedication, nitrous oxide analgesia, or IV sedation should be considered. Before prescribing or administering any of these, the patient's physician should be consulted, and the parents or caretaker informed of the change in the treatment plan. Note this informed consent procedure, as well as the reasons for the change, in the treatment plan in the record. In view of the current em-

TABLE 11–2. Potential Risk Factors

A. Dietary and Nutritional Factors
   1. Prolonged bottle feeding
   2. Special or inadequate diets
   3. Cariogenic food as behavioral reinforcers
   4. Suboptimal fluoride supplementation
B. Motor and Neurologic Factors
   1. Motor dysfunction
   2. Gross or fine motor delays or dysfunction
C. Attitudinal and Behavioral Factors
   1. Inadequate oral care procedures
   2. Crisis orientation to care
   3. Preoccupation with one's disability[13]

phasis on patient rights and the provision of treatment in the least restrictive setting, the use of physical restraint should be avoided. If restraint becomes necessary to ensure the patient's and operator's safety, the minimal and least restrictive form of restraint should be used. If restraints are required, consent should be obtained and a notation made in the patient's record. Under no circumstances should restraint be used to punish a patient. Hospitalization may be the treatment option if extensive oral surgery or restorative treatment is required for the medically compromised patient or for the patient with uncontrollable behavior problems.[22]

PREVENTIVE MEASURES AND APPROACHES

Prevention of dental disease represents a cooperative endeavor among the patient, the caretaker, and the dental team. The dental literature abounds with references to the poor oral hygiene of persons with mental retardation and suggestions for improving their dental health status. Most of the programs described were conducted as student projects in school or residential settings where coordination with dental office programs was not attempted and data were not available regarding long-term maintenance.

Dental team members are responsible for providing office-based preventive procedures, scheduling periodic recall visits, and providing the patient and caretakers with the information, materials, and skills needed to perform a home care program. When designing preventive programs for mentally retarded individuals, assessment of the person's skills, needs, and disabilities is crucial. The same toothbrushing program and educational focus is not appropriate for everyone. Risk factors for the development of dental disease should be determined. Potential risk factors are outlined in Table 11–2.

Dietary and Nutritional Factors

Children who are mentally retarded may develop carious lesions because of excessive use of cariogenic foods during bottle feeding or as behavioral reinforcers. Dietary counseling is indicated for parents and other caretakers regarding the cariogenic potential of foods, including consistency and retentiveness. Specific suggestions should be given for alternative snacks, reinforcement choices, or decreased snacking frequency (see Table 10–4). Like children with cerebral palsy, traditional snacks that include popcorn, nuts, and carrots may not be appropriate for children with chewing and swallowing problems or those on restricted diets. A discussion with the parent or caretaker will prove beneficial in outlining a realistic program. Certain dietary practices that may be cariogenic are sometimes necessary for the child's general welfare. Frequent, prolonged bottle feedings with cariogenic substances are common for children with PKU and those who fail to thrive. Dental team members will gain more parental cooperation in the long run by making suggestions such as rinsing the child's mouth with water, brushing more frequently, and supplementing with fluoride preparations rather than admonishing them to change the diet. Consultation with the child's physician or nutritionist is helpful in those instances.

Mentally retarded adults may not be exposed to nutrition education other than that received in the dental office, and they are usually receptive to dietary counseling. Mildly retarded individuals may be involved in weight reduction programs, which can provide a natural starting point of discussion for dietary counseling. Those who live in residential settings may have no control over their daily diet, but they can be taught to be discriminating when eating out or during breaks at work.

In most cases, it is impossible to accurately determine a person's fluoride history, particularly if he or she has moved from place to place. Many mentally retarded individuals may have received systemic benefits from fluoridated water and topical benefits from toothpaste, but no other topical preparations. A topical fluoride preparation is generally indicated for both children and adults if they are caries-prone. If home treatments are provided, careful monitoring is needed to avoid accidental ingestion or misuse by the patient.

Motor and Neurologic Factors

Although mental retardation primarily affects a person's ability to learn and conceptualize, motor delays and impairments are also common. Motor skills may be particularly poor, and the person may have difficulty in determining the proper placement of the toothbrush in the mouth and the bristles on the teeth and gingiva. Remembering a long sequence of steps may also be difficult. Use of repetitive verbal and physical guidance is often effective in teaching toothbrushing skills. Teaching toothbrushing techniques intraorally is generally more efficient and effective, although practice sessions with plastic models have been used in some programs. The use of a hand mirror for visual demonstration and self-monitoring is beneficial, but may be counterproductive if the person has visual-perceptual or visual-motor problems.

Oral motor dysfunction such as hyperactive gag reflexes or impaired tongue control are evident in some mentally retarded persons. Such problems can interfere with the patient's ability to tolerate or cooperate with toothbrushing, treatment procedures, or fluoride applications. The use of a brush-on fluoride gel is sometimes more successful than tray or rinse applications in such cases.

Attitudinal and Behavioral Factors

Other behaviors may interfere with effective toothbrushing. Inappropriate or excessive use of toothpaste or water are common caretaker complaints. Persons who brush too rapidly and miss areas sometimes respond to time schedules, such as the use of a kitchen timer. Persons who brush inconsistently and don't appear to be motivated need a structured program with relevant reinforcers to shape appropriate hygiene habits. Appropriate reinforcers should change when necessary according to the patient's response.

Preoccupation with one's disability and a crisis orientation to care can lead to inadequate oral hygiene or postponement of dental treatment until an emergency arises. Empathetic counseling is indicated in both situations, with an emphasis on increasing the patient's self-esteem and establishing dental health as an integral part of general health. Consultation with other community professionals such as psychologists or social workers may help in establishing continuity of care for these patients.

Community-Based Programs

The concept of home care should not be limited to procedures and education received in the dental office and at the patient's home. Many community-based programs that provide educational or vocational services for mentally retarded persons are enthusiastic about incorporating oral hygiene programs into their services. Using the approaches described in this chapter, effective oral hygiene programs can be implemented and periodically reinforced by office visits or communication with the dental team members.[12,24] When such programs are instituted in group settings, dental team members will find the following suggestions helpful to ensure continuation of the program after the initial training and implementation phase:

1. Involve the house parents, workshop supervisors, and others in the planning and implementation of the program. Supervisory staff should be responsible for monitoring the status of the program, reinforcing others who carry out the program, and training new staff members. Supervisors, therefore, need to understand all program components and their relative importance.[25]
2. Establish a practical means of communication among the supervisors, program staff, and yourself. The staff will have to

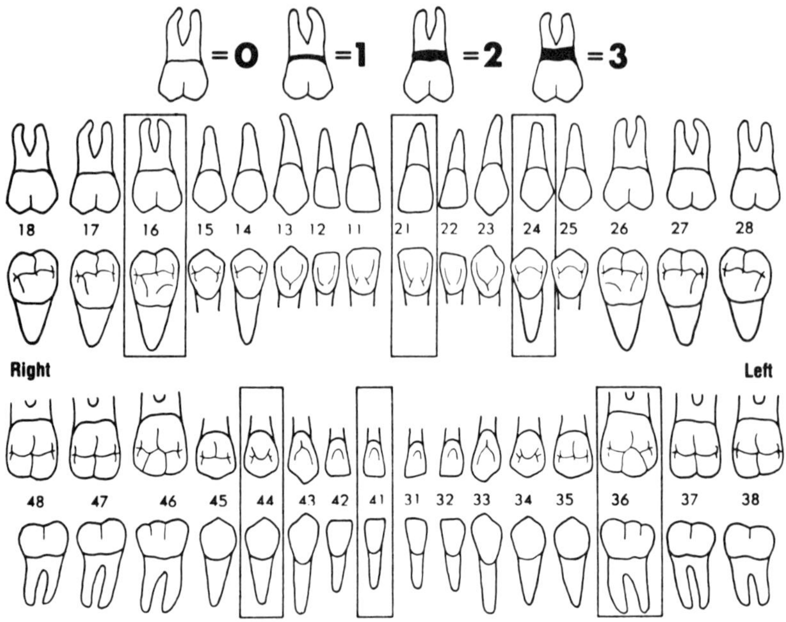

Plaque Index

0 = no debris or stain present
1 = soft debris covering less than ⅓ of the tooth surface
2 = soft debris covering over ⅓ of the tooth surface
3 = soft debris covering ⅔ or more of the tooth surface

Fig. 11–4. A modified OHI-S to monitor brushing skills.

evaluate the progress of the clients and determine whether the program is effective and appropriate. They will need your dental expertise for both. Data for oral hygiene progress (plaque removal) can be collected using disclosing solution and a standard index such as the modified OHI-S shown in Figure 11–4.[26,27] All teeth or selected teeth (those outlined) can be used to record progress.

Individualized Plans

Using this chapter as a guide, specific procedures, educational strategies, and frequency of recalls should be individualized for each patient. The preventive plan should be efficient and provide optimal benefits. Factors that may have an impact on your individualized plan for the patient include:

1. age
2. dental needs
3. mental functioning level

TABLE 11–3. Educational Approaches

Education Topic	Level of Impairment		
	Mild Mental Impairment	Moderate Impairment	Severe to Profound Impairment
Plaque	*Method*	*Method*	*Method*
Explanation of plaque	Direct primarily to patient—verbal description with visual aids and pamphlets	Describe as food that needs to be removed—use simple pictures	Counsel with caretaker
Recognition of plaque	Teach patient use of disclosing tablets	Disclosing solution applied by someone else—point out food debris	Demonstrate to caretaker
Removal of plaque	Verbal instructions supervised use of floss	Verbal—demonstration and physical assistance	Total physical assistance by caretaker
Diet			
Explanation of dietary causes of dental disease	Verbal explanation—use of visual aids and pamphlets	Pictures and simple verbal description—explain to caretaker	Explain to caretaker
Determination of food intake	Inteview patient and agree on foods list	Interview patient and caretaker. Use food models.	Interview caretaker
Counseling re: dietary habits	Verbal instructions with written instructions and pamphlets to patient	Use of food models and other visuals. Counseling also with caretaker.	Counsel with caretaker
Fluoride			
Explanation of fluoride benefits	Verbal explanation—use of visual aids and pamphlets	Use of pictures with patient. Explain to caretaker.	
Determination of fluoride intake	Verbal interview	Interview with patient and caretaker	Interview with caretaker
Application of home fluoride	Show patient mouth rinse (brush on or gel in tray)—use self-monitoring	Brush on—monitoring by caretaker	Brush on by caretaker

4. motor skills
5. living arrangements
6. caretaker cooperation and understanding
7. daily schedule
8. behavior
9. medical condition and medications
10. dietary habits
11. financial status
12. transportation

Educational Approaches

Table 11–3 outlines dental education approaches for persons with varying degrees of mental retardation. The approaches should be based on the individual's functional abilities in a variety of areas, not on his/her diagnostic classification. The amount of assistance a patient will need for home care ranges from complete independence to total assistance. If assistance is required and the patient is capable, the person providing the assistance should encourage the patient to progressively do more on his or her own. Requiring the patient to do more, while decreasing the amount of assistance given, will help to improve the patient's skill level. Guidelines that are helpful in developing and maintaining preventive programs include:

1. Involve the patient and/or caretaker as appropriate. Involvement allows the patient to participate to the extent of his or her abilities and to rehearse the skills being taught, and it provides the caretaker with an understanding of his or her role.
2. Whenever possible, provide a means for checking for plaque control.
3. Use terminology the patient and caretaker can understand. Remember, simplification of language does not necessitate the use of a sing-song childish tone of voice with mentally retarded adults.
4. Go slowly. Teach one concept or step at a time. Ask the patient and/or caretaker to repeat or demonstrate the concept or step before proceeding to the next step. When teaching toothbrushing, the removal of plaque is more important than the actual toothbrushing technique.
5. Remember to give verbal praise and positively reinforce the patient in other ways.
6. End the session on a positive note. If the patient becomes tired, restless, or inattentive, review the last successfully

completed step before dismissing the patient.

7. During subsequent visits, review steps or activities from the previous appointment, reinforcing what the patient remembers while demonstrating and repeating what the patient omits.
8. Encourage the patient and/or caretaker to practice what has been learned. Decrease their reliance on dental professionals for monitoring and maintenance of oral hygiene.

PATIENT SCENARIOS

Patient 1

Description

Debbie is a 12-year-old child with Down's syndrome who has lived in six different foster homes. She has received dental care sporadically and is coming to your office for an examination. Her caseworker will be bringing her for the appointment.

Anticipated Patient Needs

—thorough oral examination
—oral hygiene instructions
—radiographs
—limited dental treatment

Awareness Strategies

1. What information should you discuss with the caseworker prior to the appointment about Debbie's handicapping condition?
2. What other handicapping conditions or medical problems could Debbie have that you need to know about?
3. How would you approach home care instructions in this case?
4. How can you ensure continuity of care with Debbie?

Patient 2

Description

Michelle is a two-year-old youngster with severe mental retardation and multiple congenital anomalies and medical problems. During dental screening at an early intervention program, you noted that she had extensive dental caries and abscesses as a result of prolonged, excessive bottle feeding. Her mother wants her to receive dental treatment through your office.

Anticipated Patient Needs

—complete examination
—full mouth radiographs
—extractions, crowns, and space maintainers
—dietary and oral hygiene counseling
—physician's consultation

Awareness Strategies

1. What preliminary information do you need about her conditions prior to treatment?
2. What might be the most appropriate treatment setting for Michelle?
3. What preventive instructions and procedures should be taught to Michelle's mother?
4. What procedures and processes would you use to involve the parent during the recall appointment?

Patient 3

Description

John is a 26-year-old moderately mentally retarded man who lives in a group home and attends a work activity program. His counselor will bring him to the first appointment, but he will take the bus by himself to subsequent appointments. He received regular dental care in a residential home, but is now seeking care in your office.

Anticipated Patient Needs

—thorough examination
—specific radiographs
—debridement and prophylaxis
—oral care instructions
—minimal treatment

Awareness Strategies

1. What factors might impinge on appointment scheduling and treatment planning?
2. What minor management problems might you encounter?
3. Describe an approach to oral hygiene instruction with John, including measures for self-monitoring.
4. What mechanisms would be useful for facilitating patient scheduling and payment?

REFERENCES

1. Grossman, H. (ed.): Manual on Terminology and Classification in Mental Retardation. A.A.M.D. Special Publication Series No. 2. Baltimore, Garamond Pridemark Press, 1973.
2. Robinson, H., and Robinson, M.: The Mentally Retarded Child: A Psychological Approach. New York, McGraw-Hill, 1965.
3. Baroff, G.: Mental Retardation: Nature, Cause and Management. Washington, D.C., Hemisphere Publishing, 1974.
4. Drew, C., Handman, M., and Blum, H.: Mental Retardation: Social and Educational Perspectives. St. Louis, C.V. Mosby, 1977.
5. Neisworth, J.T., and Smith, R.: Retardation: Issues, Assessments and Intervention. New York, McGraw-Hill, 1978.
6. Craft, M.: Classification, criteria, epidemiology and causation. *In* Trendgold's Mental Retardation. Edited by M. Craft. London, Bailliere Tindall, 1979.
7. Ingalls, R.P.: Mental Retardation: The Changing Outlook. New York, John Wiley & Sons, 1978.
8. Martin, R.: Legal regulation of services to the developmentally disabled. *In* Current Trends for the Developmentally Disabled. Edited by M.S. Berkler et al. Baltimore, University Park Press, 1978.
9. Craft, M., and Harper, P.: Primary genetic disorders and their management. *In* Trendgold's Mental Retardation. Edited by M. Craft. London, Bailliere Tindall, 1979.
10. Capute, A.: Developmental disabilities. Dent. Clin. North Am. *18*:3, July, 1974.
11. Douglas, C.P., and Holt, K.J. (eds.): Mental Retardation: Prenatal Diagnosis and Infant Assessment. London, Butterworth and Co., 1972.
12. Nowak, A.J.: Dentistry for the Handicapped Patient. St. Louis, C.V. Mosby, 1976.
13. Entwistle, B., and Casamassimo, P.: Assessing dental health problems of children with developmental disabilities. J. Behav. Pediatr., *2*(3):115–121, 1981.
14. Brown, J.P., and Schodel, D.R.: A review of controlled surveys of dental disease in handicapped persons. J. Dent. Child., *43*:17–24, 1976.
15. Tesini, D.A.: An annotated review of the literature of dental caries and periodontal disease in mentally retarded individuals. Special Care in Dent. *1*:75–87, 1981
16. Snyder, J.R., Knopp, J.J., and Jordan, W.A.: Dental problems of non-institutionalized mentally retarded children. Northwest Dent., *39*:123–33, 1960.
17. Cohen, H.J., and Diner, H.: The significance of developmental dental defects in neurological diagnosis. Pediatrics, *46*:737–47, 1970.
18. Via, W.F., and Churchill, M.D.: Relationships of enamel hypoplasia to abnormal events of gestation and birth. J. Am. Dent. Assoc., *59*:702–707, 1957.
19. Jorgenson, R., Levin, L., and McKusick, U.: Heritable oral handicaps. Dent. Clin. North Am. *18*:3, July, 1974.
20. Stewart, R.E., et al.: Pediatric Dentistry. St. Louis, C.V. Mosby, 1982.
21. Nowak, A.J., (ed): Radiology in pediatric dentistry. Pediatric Dentistry, January, 1982. Monograph of Proceedings of Conference on Radiographic Exposure in Pediatric Dentistry, Cincinnati, Ohio, April, 1981.
22. Snow, M., and Stiefel, D.: Dental Treatment of the Mentally Retarded Patient. Project DECOD (Dental Education for Care of the Disabled). School of Dentistry, University of Washington, 1978.
23. Wexler, D.: Behavior modification and other behavioral change procedures: the emerging law and the proposed Florida guidelines. *In* Current Trends for the Developmentally Disabled. Edited by M.S. Berkler, et al. Baltimore, University Park Press, 1978.
24. Casamassimo, P.S., and Nowak, A.J.: Planning a preventive dentistry program

for the handicapped patient in an intermediate facility. Rehab. Lit, 38(8):251–257, 1977.
25. Lange, B., and Rhodes, J.: Investigation of alternative approaches to the acquisition of oral hygiene skills for the developmentally retarded. J. Prevent. Dent., 6:297–302, 1980.
26. Darby, M.L. and Bauer, D.M.: Research Methods for Oral Health Professionals. St. Louis, C.V. Mosby, 1980.
27. Lange, B.: The Effects of Modeling in the Oral Health Care of Mentally Retarded. Unpublished doctoral dissertation. Lincoln, University of Nebraska, 1980.

INDEX